Erwin Dee Kord (Ed.)

Spontaneous Cerebrospinal Fluid Leak

Erwin Dee Kord (Ed.)

Spontaneous Cerebrospinal Fluid Leak

Spinal, Cord, Fluid, Leak, Syndrome, Medical, Brain

Solv

Publisher:
Solv is a trademark of
International Book Market Service Ltd., 17 Rue Meldrum, Beau Bassin, 1713-01 Mauritius
Email: info@bookmarketservice.com
Website: www.bookmarketservice.com

Published in 2012

Printed in: U.S.A., U.K., Germany. This book was not produced in Mauritius.

ISBN: 978-613-8-69292-8

Contents

Articles

Spontaneous cerebrospinal fluid leak 1

Cerebrospinal fluid 10

Dura mater 16

Meninges 20

Cerebrospinal fluid leak 22

Idiopathic 22

Facial weakness 24

Epidural blood patch 25

Georg Schaltenbrand 26

Spinal canal 27

Orthostatic headache 28

Dysgeusia 29

Subdural effusion 39

Neurological disorders 39

References

Article Sources and Contributors 44

Image Sources, Licenses and Contributors 45

Spontaneous cerebrospinal fluid leak

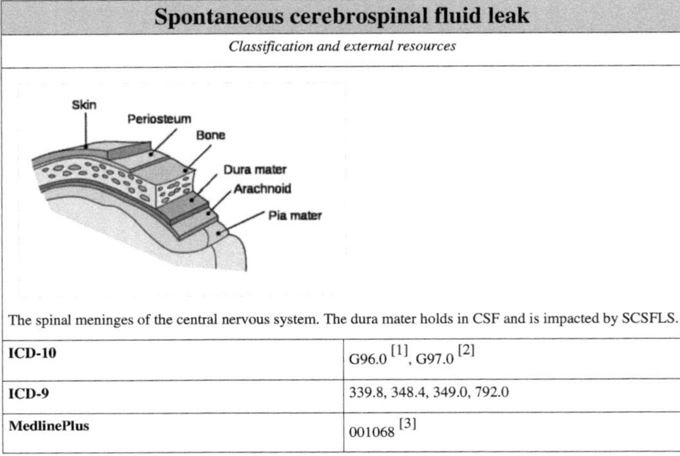

Spontaneous cerebrospinal fluid leak	
Classification and external resources	
The spinal meninges of the central nervous system. The dura mater holds in CSF and is impacted by SCSFLS.	
ICD-10	G96.0 [1], G97.0 [2]
ICD-9	339.8, 348.4, 349.0, 792.0
MedlinePlus	001068 [3]

Spontaneous cerebrospinal fluid leak syndrome (SCSFLS) is a medical condition in which the cerebrospinal fluid (CSF) held in and around a human brain and spinal cord leaks out of the surrounding protective sac, the dura, for no apparent reason. The dura, a tough, inflexible tissue, is the outermost of the three layers of the meninges, the system of meninges surrounding the brain and spinal cord. (The other two meningeal layers are the pia mater and the arachnoid mater).

A spontaneous cerebrospinal fluid leak is one of several types of cerebrospinal fluid leaks and occurs due to the presence of one or more holes in the dura. A *spontaneous* CSF leak, as opposed to traumatically caused CSF leaks, arises idiopathically. A loss of CSF greater than its rate of production leads to a decreased volume inside the skull known as intracranial hypotension. A CSF leak is most often characterized by a severe and disabling headache and a spectrum of various symptoms which occur as a result of ICH. These symptoms can include: dizziness, nausea, fatigue, a metallic taste in the mouth (indicative of a cranial leak), myoclonus, tinnitus, tingling in the limbs, facial weakness amongst others. A CT scan can identify the site of a cerebrospinal fluid leakage. Once identified, the leak can often be repaired by an epidural blood patch, an injection of the patient's own blood at the site of the leak.

SCSFLS afflicts 5 out of every 100,000 people. On average, the condition is developed at the age of 42, and women are twice as likely as men to develop the condition. Some people with SCSFLS chronically leak cerebrospinal fluid despite repeated attempts at patching, leading to long-term disability due to pain and nerve damage. SCSFLS was first described by German neurologist Georg Schaltenbrand in 1938 and by American physician Henry Woltman of the Mayo Clinic in the 1950s.

Classification

SCSFLS is classified into two main types, cranial leaks[4] and spinal leaks.[5] Cranial leaks occur in the head. In some cases, CSF can be seen dripping out of the nose,[6] [7] or ear.[4] Spinal leaks occur when one or more holes form in the dura along the spinal cord.[5] Both cranial and spinal spontaneous CSF leaks cause neurological symptoms as well as spontaneous intracranial hypotension, diminished volume and pressure of the cranium.[8] While referred to as *intracranial hypotension* the intracranial pressure may be normal, but low-volume CSF is instead the underlying issue. For this reason SCSFLS is referred to as *CSF hypovolemia* as opposed to *CSF hypotension*.[9] [10]

[11] [12]

Signs and symptoms

Symptoms resulting from nerve impact[13]

Nerve	Function	Symptoms
optic (2)	optic nerve crossing	blurred vision
chorda tympani (Branch of 7)	taste	taste distortion
facial (7)	facial nerve	facial weakness and numbness
vestibulocochlear (8)	hearing, balance	hearing and balance problems
glossopharyngeal (9)	taste	taste distortion

Most people who develop SCSFLS feel a sudden onset of a severe and acute headache.[12] [14] It is an orthostatic headache, in which the pain is worse when the patient is vertical and less severe when horizontal.[15] Other symptoms include severe dizziness and vertigo, facial numbness or weakness, double vision, fatigue, a metallic taste in the mouth, nausea, and vomiting.[12] Leaking CSF can sometimes be observed as discharge through the nose or ear.[16] Orthostatic headaches can be incapacitating;[17] [18] these symptoms can be sufficiently disabling to make those afflicted unable to work.[12] [18] [19] Some patients with CSF leak will develop headaches that begin in the afternoon. This is known as *second-half-of-the-day headache*. This may be the initial presentation of CSF leak or appear after treatment and likely indicates a slow CSF leak.[20]

Lack of CSF pressure and volume allows the brain to descend through the foramen magnum, or occipital bone, the large opening at the base of the skull. The lower portion of the brain is believed to stretch or impact one or more cranial nerve complexes, thereby causing a variety of sensory symptoms. Nerves that can be affected and their related symptoms are detailed in the table at right.[12] [13] [19]

Causes

The two main theories as to the underlying cause of SCSFLS are as a result of a connective tissue disorder or spinal drainage problems.

Connective Tissue Theory

A spontaneous CSF leak is idiopathic; it can arise spontaneously or from an unknown cause.[19] [21] Various scientists and physicians have suggested that this condition may be the result of an underlying connective tissue disorder affecting the spinal dura.[12] [13] [22] [23] It may also run in families and be associated with aortic aneurysms and joint hypermobility.[13] [24] Up to two thirds of those afflicted demonstrate some type of generalized connective tissue disorder.[13] [23] Marfan syndrome, Ehlers-Danlos syndrome and autosomal dominant polycystic kidney disease are the three most common connective tissue disorders associated with SCSFLS.[13]

Roughly 20% of patients with SCSFLS exhibit features of Marfan syndrome, including tall stature, chest divot (pectus excavatum), joint hypermobility and arched palate. However these patients do not exhibit any other Marfan syndrome presentations.[13]

Spinal Drainage Theory

Some other studies have proposed that issues with the spinal venous drainage system may cause a CSF leak.[25] According to this theory, dural holes and intracranial hypotension are symptoms caused by low pressure in the epidural space due to outflow to the heart through the inferior vena cava vein.[25]

Other causes

Patients with a nude (absent) nerve root are at increased risk for developing recurrent CSF leaks.[26] Cranial CSF leaks are as a result of intracranial hypertension in a vast majority of cases. The increased pressure causes a rupture of the cranial dura mater, leading to CSF leak and intracranial hypotension.[27] [28] Lumbar disc herniation has been reported to cause CSF leak in at least one case.[29] Degenerative spinal disc diseases cause a disc to pierce the dura mater, leading to a CSF leak.[13]

Another view of the cause of orthostatic headaches proposes a malformed distribution of craniospinal elasticity as a result of the collapse of the lower spine's CSF space resulting in the collapse of the dura sac.[13]

Pathophysiology

Cerebrospinal fluid is produced by the choroid plexus in the brain and contained by the dura and arachnoid layers of the meninges.[12] [22] [30] The brain floats in CSF, which also transports nutrients to the brain and spinal cord. As holes form in the spinal dura mater, CSF leaks out into the surrounding space. The CSF is then absorbed into the spinal epidural venous plexus or soft tissues around the spine.[13] [31] Due to the sterile conditions of the soft tissues around the spine there is no risk of meningitis.[13]

Diagnosis

The primary place of first complaint to a physician is a hospital emergency room.[14] [32] Up to 94% of those suffering from SCSFLS are initially misdiagnosed. Incorrect diagnoses include migraines, meningitis, and psychiatric disorders. The average time from onset of symptoms until definitive diagnosis is 13 months.[33] A study found a 0% success rate for proper diagnosis in the emergency department.[32]

Diagnosis of CSF leak can be done through various imaging techniques or chemical tests. The use of CT, MRI and assays are the most common types of CSF leak tests.

CT

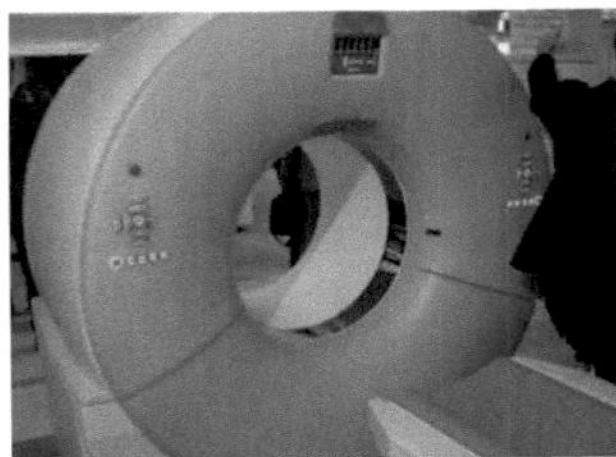

A typical CT scan machine used in the imaging and diagnosis of spinal fluid leak by using non-ionic contrast

Diagnosis of a cerebrospinal fluid leak is performed through a combination of measurement of the CSF pressure and a computed tomography myelogram (CTM) scan of the spinal column for fluid leaks.[13] The opening fluid pressure in the spinal canal is obtained by performing a lumbar puncture, also known as a spinal tap. Once the pressure is measured, radiopaque contrast material is injected into the spinal fluid. The contrast then diffuses out through the dura sac before leaking through dural holes. This allows for a CTM with fluoroscopy to locate and image any sites of dura rupture via contrast seen outside the dura sac in the imagery.[12] [16] [22]

MRI

Magnetic resonance imaging is historically less effective at directly imaging sites of CSF leak. MRI studies may show pachymeningeal enhancement (when the dura mater looks thick and inflamed) and an Arnold-Chiari malformation many, but not all, cases.[13] An Arnold-Chiari malformation occurs when the brain sags and has a downward displacement due to the decreased volume and buoyancy of cerebrospinal fluid in which the brain floats.[13] MRIs can present as completely normal, however, and are not the study of choice.[13] [22] An alternate method of locating the site of a CSF leak is to use heavily T2-weighted MR myelography.[13] This has been effective in identifying the sites of a CSF leak without the need for a CT scan, lumbar puncture, and contrast and at locating fluid collections such as CSF pooling.[34] MRIs done on patients sitting upright demonstrated no difference in MRI results compared to those lying down.[32] The use of intrathecal contrast and MR Meyrlography is also an alternative method of locating CSF leaks with a very high degree of success.[13]

Assay

When cranial CSF leak is suspected because of discharge from the nose or ear that is potentially CSF, the fluid can be collected and tested with a beta-2 transferrin assay.[35] This test can positively identify if the fluid is cerebrospinal fluid.[35]

CSF analysis

Patients with CSF leak have been noted to have very low or even negative opening pressures. However, patients with confirmed CSF leaks may also demonstrate completely normal opening pressures. In 18–46% of cases, the CSF pressure is measured within the normal range.[13] [36] [37] [38] Analysis of spinal fluid may demonstrate lymphocytic pleocytosis and elevated protein content or xanthochromia. This is hypothesized to be due to increased permeability of dilated meningeal blood vessels and a decrease of CSF flow in the lumbar subarachnoid space.[13]

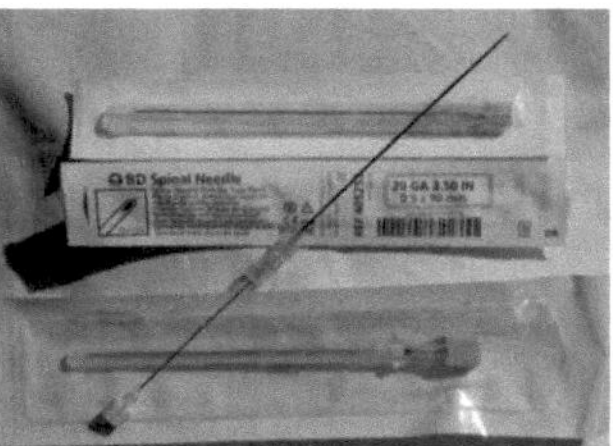

Spinal needles used in lumbar puncture and introduction of contrast into the spine

Clinical presentation

The diagnostic criteria for SCSFLS is based on the 2004 International Classification of Headache Disorders, 2nd edn (ICHD-II) (Table 1) (50) criteria. However, the presentation of patients with confirmed diagnosis may be very different from that of the clinical diagnostic criteria and cannot be considered authoritative.[13]

Treatment

Epidural Blood Patch

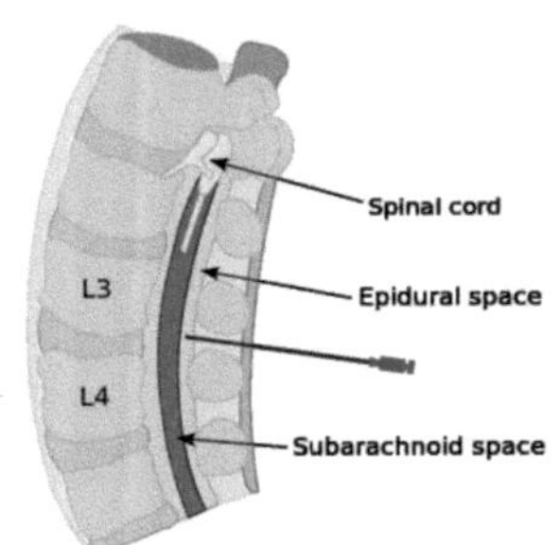

The epidural syringe is filled with autologous blood and injected in the epidural space in order to close holes in the dura mater.

The treatment of choice for this condition is the surgical application of epidural blood patches,[17] [39] [40] which has a 90% success rate in treating dural holes;[19] [41] a rate higher than that of a conservative treatment of bed rest and hydration.[42] Through the injection of a person's own blood into the area of the hole in the dura, an epidural blood patch uses blood's clotting factors to clot the sites of holes. The volume of autologous blood and number of patch attempts for patients is highly variable.[17] One quarter to one third of SCSFLS patients do not have relief of symptoms from epidural blood patching.[13]

Fibrin glue sealant

If blood patches alone do not succeed in closing the dural tears, placement of percutaneous fibrin glue can be used in place of blood patching, raising the effectiveness of forming a clot and arresting CSF leakage.[5] [13] [13] [43]

Surgical drain technique

In extreme cases of intractable CSF leak, a surgical lumbar drain has been used.[44] [45] [46] This procedure is believed to decrease spinal CSF volume while increasing intracranial CSF pressure and volume.[44] This procedure restores normal intracranial CSF volume and pressure while promoting the healing of dural tears by lowering the pressure and volume in the dura.[44] [46] This procedure has led to positive results leading to relief of symptoms for up to one year.[44] [45]

Neurosurgical repair

For patients who do not respond to either epidural blood patching or fibrin glue, neurosurgery is available to directly repair leaking meningeal diverticula. The areas of dura leak can be tied together in a process called ligation and then a metal clip can be placed in order to hold the ligation closed.[13] Alternatively, a small compress called a muscle pledget can be placed over the dura leak and then sealed with gel foam and fibrin glue.[13] Primary suturing is rarely able to repair a CSF leak and in some patients exploration of the dura may be required to properly locate all sites of CSF leak.[13]

Other treatments

The use of an abdominal binder has also been employed as a treatment.[13]

Prognosis

Final outcomes for people with SCSFLS remain poorly studied.[13] Some of those afflicted continue to leak CSF from one or more sites and may suffer from unremitting symptoms for many years.[12] [22] [47] People with chronic SCSFLS may be disabled and unable to work.[13] [] Recurrent CSF leak at an alternate site after recent repair is common.[48]

Complications

Several complications can occur as a result of SCSFLS including decreased cranial pressure, brain herniation, infection, blood pressure problems, transient paralysis, and coma.The primary and most serious complication of SCSFLS is spontaneous intracranial hypotension, where pressure in the brain is severely decreased.[12] [22] [49] This complication leads to the hallmark symptom of severe orthostatic headaches.[13] [49]

People with cranial CSF leaks have a higher chance of developing meningitis than those with spinal CSF leaks.[35] Additionally, if cranial leaks last more than seven days, the chances of developing meningitis are significantly higher.[35] Spinal CSF leaks do not usually result in meningitis due to the mostly aseptic conditions of the spinal dura.[35] When a CSF leak occurs at the temporal bone surgery becomes necessary in order to prevent infection and repair the leak.[50] Orthostatic hypotension is another complication which occurs due to autonomic dysfunction when blood pressure drops significantly.[47] The autonomic dysfunction is caused by compression of the brain stem, which controls breathing and circulation.[47]

An Arnold-Chiari malformation is a downward displacement of lower parts of the brain through the skull opening that occurs due to a lack of CSF volume and pressure. A further, albeit rare, complication of CSF leak is transient quadriplegia due to a sudden and significant loss of CSF. This loss results in hindbrain herniation and causes major compression of the upper cervical spinal cord. The quadriplegia dissipates once the patient lays supine.[51] [51] An extremely rare complication of SCSFLS is third nerve palsy, where the ability to move one's eyes becomes difficult and interrupted due to compression of the third cranial nerve.[52]

There are documented cases of reversible dementia and coma.[53] Coma due to a CSF leak has been successfully treated by using blood patches and/or fibrin glue and placing the patient in the Trendelenburg position.[54] Empty sella syndrome, a boney structure that surround the pituitary gland, occurs in CSF leak patients.[27] [55]

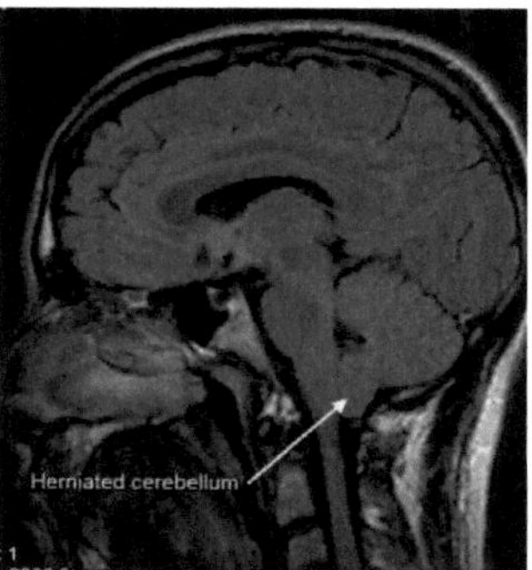

Arnold-Chiari malformation is a complication of spontaneous CSF leak, where brain tissue moves down through the opening at the base of the skull due to low volume and pressure of CSF

Epidemiology

A 1994 community-based study indicated that two out of every 100,000 people suffered from SCSFLS, while a 2004 emergency room-based study indicated five per 100,000.[13] [22] SCSFLS generally affects the young and middle aged;[44] the average age for onset is 42.3 years, but onset can range from ages 22 to 61.[56] In an 11-year study women were found to be twice as likely to be affected as men.[57] [58]

Studies have shown that SCSFLS runs in families and it is suspected that genetic similarity in families includes weakness in the dura mater, which leads to SCSFLS.[13] [59] Large scale population-based studies have not yet been conducted.[22] While a majority of SCSFLS cases continue to be undiagnosed or misdiagnosed, an actual increase in occurrence is unlikely.[22]

History

Spontaneous CSF leaks have been described by notable physicians and reported in medical journals dating back to the early 1900s.[60] [61] German neurologist Georg Schaltenbrand reported in 1938 and 1953 what he termed "aliquorrhea", a condition marked by very low, unobtainable, or even negative CSF pressures. The symptoms included orthostatic headaches and other features that are now recognized as spontaneous intracranial hypotension. A few decades earlier, the same syndrome had been described in French literature as "hypotension of spinal fluid" and "ventricular collapse". In 1940, Henry Woltman of the Mayo Clinic wrote about "headaches associated with decreased intracranial pressure". The full clinical manifestations of intracranial hypotension and CSF leaks were described in several publications reported between the 1960s and early 1990s.[61] Modern reports of spontaneous CSF leak have been reported to medical journals since the late 1980s.[62]

Research and experimental treatments

IV Cosyntropin, a corticosteroid that causes the brain to produce additional spinal fluid to replace the volume of the lost CSF and alleviate symptoms, has been used to treat CSF leaks.[63] [64]

In two small studies of two patients and another with one patient who suffered from recurrent CSF leaks where repeated blood patches failed to form clots and relieve symptoms, the patients received temporary but complete resolution of symptoms with an epidural saline infusion.[65] [66] The saline infusion temporarily restores the volume necessary for a patient to avoid SIH until the leak can be repaired properly.[13] Intrathecal saline infusion is used in urgent cases such as intractable pain or decreased consciousness.[13]

The gene TGFBR2 has been implicated in several connective tissue disorders including Marfan syndrome, arterial tortuosity and thoracic aortic aneurysm. A study of patients with SCSFLS demonstrated no mutations in this gene.[13] Minor features of Marfan syndrome has been found in 20% of CSF leak patients. Abnormal findings of fibrillin-1 has been documented in these CSF leak patients but only one patient demonstrated a fibrillin-1 defect consistent with Marfan syndrome.[13] [67]

See also

- Subdural effusion

References

[1] http://apps.who.int/classifications/icd10/browse/2010/en#/G96.0

[2] http://apps.who.int/classifications/icd10/browse/2010/en#/G97.0

[3] http://www.nlm.nih.gov/medlineplus/ency/article/001068.htm

[4] Lloyd, K. M.; Delgaudio, J. M.; Hudgins, P. A. (2008). "Imaging of Skull Base Cerebrospinal Fluid Leaks in Adults". *Radiology* **248** (3): 725. doi:10.1148/radiol.2483070362. PMID 18710972.

[5] Gordon, N. (2009). "Spontaneous intracranial hypotension". *Developmental Medicine & Child Neurology* **51** (12): 932–935. doi:10.1111/j.1469-8749.2009.03514.x. PMID 19909307.

[6] Wise, S. K.; Schlosser, R. J. (2007). "Evaluation of spontaneous nasal cerebrospinal fluid leaks". *Current Opinion in Otolaryngology & Head and Neck Surgery* **15** (1): 28–34. doi:10.1097/MOO.0b013e328011bc76. PMID 17211180.

[7] Hayek, S. M.; Fattouh, M.; Dews, T.; Kapural, L.; Malak, O.; Mekhail, N. (2003). "Successful treatment of spontaneous cerebrospinal fluid leak headache with fluoroscopically guided epidural blood patch: a report of four cases". *Pain medicine (Malden, Mass.)* **4** (4): 373–378. doi:10.1111/j.1526-4637.2003.03037.x. PMID 14750917.

[8] Maher, CO; Meyer; Mokri (2000). "Surgical treatment of spontaneous spinal cerebrospinal fluid leaks". *Neurosurgical focus* **9** (1): e7. doi:10.3171/foc.2000.9.1.7. PMID 16859268.

[9] Greenberg, Mark (2006). *Handbook of neurosurgery* (http://books.google.com/?id=ExHcxxufG8sC&pg=PA178&dq=Spontaneous+intracranial+hypotension&cd=1#v=onepage&q=Spontaneous intracranial hypotension). New York, NY: Thieme Medical Publishers. p. 178.

ISBN 0865779090. . Retrieved 18 December 2009.

[10] Neil R. Miller; William Fletcher Hoyt (2005). *Walsh and Hoyt's clinical neuro-ophthalmology* (http://books.google.com/ books?id=ATTlVWi3mvwC&pg=PA1303). Lippincott Williams & Wilkins. pp. 1303–. ISBN 9780781748117. . Retrieved 8 November 2010.

[11] Mokri, B. (1999). "Spontaneous cerebrospinal fluid leaks: from intracranial hypotension to cerebrospinal fluid hypovolemia--evolution of a concept". *Mayo Clinic proceedings. Mayo Clinic* **74** (11): 1113–1123. doi:10.4065/74.11.1113. PMID 10560599.

[12] Schievink, WI (2000). "Spontaneous spinal cerebrospinal fluid leaks: a review". *Neurosurgical focus* **9** (1): e8. doi:10.3171/foc.2000.9.1.8. PMID 16859269.

[13] Schievink, W. I. (2008). "Spontaneous spinal cerebrospinal fluid leaks". *Cephalalgia : an international journal of headache* **28** (12): 1345–1356. doi:10.1111/j.1468-2982.2008.01776.x. PMID 19037970.

[14] Vaidhyanath, R.; Kenningham, R.; Khan, A.; Messios, N. (2007). "Spontaneous intracranial hypotension: a cause of severe acute headache". *Emergency Medicine Journal* **24** (10): 739–741. doi:10.1136/emj.2007.048694. PMC 2658456. PMID 17901290.

[15] Schievink, W.; Palestrant, D.; Maya, M.; Rappard, G. (2009). "Spontaneous spinal cerebrospinal fluid leak as a cause of coma after craniotomy for clipping of an unruptured intracranial aneurysm". *Journal of neurosurgery* **110** (3): 521–524. doi:10.3171/2008.9.JNS08670. PMID 19012477.

[16] Hofmann, E.; Behr, R.; Schwager, K. (2009). "Imaging of cerebrospinal fluid leaks". *Klinische Neuroradiologie* **19** (2): 111–121. doi:10.1007/s00062-009-9008-x. PMID 19636501.

[17] Mehta, B.; Tarshis, J. (2009). "Repeated large-volume epidural blood patches for the treatment of spontaneous intracranial hypotension". *Canadian Journal of Anesthesia/Journal canadien d'anesthésie* **56** (8): 609. doi:10.1007/s12630-009-9121-y. PMID 19495908.

[18] Mea, E.; Chiapparini, L.; Savoiardo, M.; Franzini, A.; Bussone, G.; Leone, M. (2009). "Clinical features and outcomes in spontaneous intracranial hypotension: a survey of 90 consecutive patients". *Neurological Sciences* **30** (S1): 11. doi:10.1007/s10072-009-0060-8. PMID 19415418.

[19] Victor, Maurice; Ropper, Allan H.; Adams, Raymond Delacy; Brown, Robert F. (2005). *Adams and Victor's principles of neurology.* New York: McGraw-Hill Medical Pub. Division. pp. 541–543. ISBN 0-07-141620-X.

[20] Leep Hunderfund, A. N.; Mokri, B. (2011). "Second-half-of-the-day headache as a *manifestation of* spontaneous CSF leak". *Journal of Neurology.* doi:10.1007/s00415-011-6181-z. PMID 21811806.

[21] Schievink, W. I.; Louy, C. (2007). "Precipitating Factors of Spontaneous Spinal Csf Leaks and Intracranial Hypotension". *Neurology* **69**: 700. doi:10.1212/01.wnl.0000267324.68013.8e.

[22] Schievink, W. I. (2006). "Spontaneous Spinal Cerebrospinal Fluid Leaks and Intracranial Hypotension". *Journal of the American Medical Association* **295** (19): 2286. doi:10.1001/jama.295.19.2286. PMID 16705110.

[23] Liu, F. -C.; Fuh, J. -L.; Wang, Y. -F.; Wang, S. -J. (2011). "Connective tissue disorders in *patients with* spontaneous intracranial hypotension". *Cephalalgia* **31** (6): 691–695. doi:10.1177/0333102410394676. PMID 21220378.

[24] Mokri, B. (2007). "Familial Occurrence of Spontaneous Spinal CSF Leaks: Underlying Connective Tissue Disorder (CME)". *Headache: the Journal of Head and Face Pain* **48**: 146. doi:10.1111/j.1526-4610.2007.00979.x.

[25] Franzini, A.; Messina, G.; Nazzi, V.; Mea, E.; Leone, M.; Chiapparini, L.; Broggi, G.; Bussone, G. (2009). "Spontaneous intracranial hypotension syndrome: a novel speculative physiopathological hypothesis and a novel patch method in a series of 28 consecutive patients". *Journal of neurosurgery* **112** (2): 090710065136044. doi:10.3171/2009.6.JNS09415. PMID 19591547.

[26] Schievink, WI; Jacques, L (2003). "Recurrent spontaneous spinal cerebrospinal fluid leak associated with "nude nerve root" syndrome: case report". *Neurosurgery* **53** (5): 1216–8; discussion 1218–9. doi:10.1227/01.NEU.0000089483.30857.11. PMID 14580290.

[27] Woodworth, B. A.; Palmer, J. N. (2009). "Spontaneous cerebrospinal fluid leaks". *Current Opinion in Otolaryngology & Head and Neck Surgery* **17** (1): 59. doi:10.1097/MOO.0b013e3283200017. PMID 19225307.

[28] Schlosser, RJ; Wilensky, EM; Grady, MS; Bolger, WE (2003). "Elevated intracranial pressures in spontaneous cerebrospinal fluid leaks". *American journal of rhinology* **17** (4): 191–5. PMID 12962187.

[29] Kim, K. T.; Kim, Y. B. (2010). "Spontaneous Intracranial Hypotension Secondary to Lumbar Disc Herniation". *Journal of Korean Neurosurgical Society* **47** (1): 48. doi:10.3340/jkns.2010.47.1.48. PMC 2817515. PMID 20157378.

[30] Michael Schuenke; Udo Schumacher; Erik Schulte; Edward D. Lamperti, Lawrence M. Ross (2007). *Head and neuroanatomy* (http:// books.google.com/books?id=Y0-Rf_m7xj4C). Thieme. ISBN 9783131421012. . Retrieved 8 November 2010.

[31] Inamasu, J.; Guiot, B. (2006). "Intracranial hypotension with spinal pathology". *The Spine Journal* **6** (5): 591. doi:10.1016/j.spinee.2005.12.026. PMID 16934734.

[32] Schievink, W. I.; Maya, M. M.; Moser, F.; Tourje, J.; Torbati, S. (2007). "Frequency of spontaneous intracranial hypotension in the emergency department". *The Journal of Headache and Pain* **8** (6): 325. doi:10.1007/s10194-007-0421-8. PMID 18071632.

[33] Schievink, W. I. (2003). "Misdiagnosis of Spontaneous Intracranial Hypotension". *Archives of Neurology* **60** (12): 1713. doi:10.1001/archneur.60.12.1713. PMID 14676045.

[34] Wang, Y. -F.; Lirng, J. -F.; Fuh, J. -L.; Hseu, S. -S.; Wang, S. -J. (2009). "Heavily T2-weighted MR myelography vs CT myelography in spontaneous intracranial hypotension". *Neurology* **73** (22): 1892. doi:10.1212/WNL.0b013e3181c3fd99. PMID 19949036.

[35] Abuabara, A (2007). "Cerebrospinal fluid rhinorrhoea: diagnosis and management". *Medicina oral, patologia oral y cirugia bucal* **12** (5): E397–400. PMID 17767107.

[36] Kelley, G (2004). "CSF hypovolemia vs intracranial hypotension in "spontaneous intracranial hypotension syndrome"". *Neurology* **62** (8): 1453. PMID 15111706.

[37]　Canas, N; Medeiros, E; Fonseca, AT; Palma-Mira, F (2004). "CSF volume loss in spontaneous intracranial hypotension". *Neurology* **63** (1): 186–7. PMID 15249640.

[38]　Mark S. Greenberg (2006). *Handbook of neurosurgery* (http://books.google.com/books?id=ExHcxxufG8sC&pg=PA178). Thieme. pp. 178–. ISBN 9783131108869. . Retrieved 8 November 2010.

[39]　Peng, PW; Farb (2008). "Spontaneous C1-2 CSF leak treated with high cervical epidural blood patch". *The Canadian journal of neurological sciences. Le journal canadien des sciences neurologiques* **35** (1): 102–5. PMID 18380287.

[40]　Grimaldi, D.; Mea, E.; Chiapparini, L.; Ciceri, E.; Nappini, S.; Savoiardo, M.; Castelli, M.; Cortelli, P. et al. (2004). "Spontaneous low cerebrospinal pressure: a mini review". *Neurological Sciences* **25** (S3): s135. doi:10.1007/s10072-004-0272-x. PMID 15549523.

[41]　Kessler, P.; Wulf, H. (2008). "Duraperforation - postpunktioneller Kopfschmerz - Prophylaxe- und Therapiemöglichkeiten". *AINS - Anästhesiologie · Intensivmedizin · Notfallmedizin · Schmerztherapie* **43** (5): 346. doi:10.1055/s-2008-1079107. PMID 18464211.

[42]　Wang, S.; Lirng, J.; Hseu, S.; Chan, K. (2008). "Spontaneous Intracranial Hypotension Treated by Epidural Blood Patches". *Acta Anaesthesiologica Taiwanica* **46** (3): 129–133. doi:10.1016/S1875-4597(08)60007-7. PMID 18809524.

[43]　Schievink, W. I.; Maya, M. M.; Moser, F. M. (2004). "Treatment of spontaneous intracranial hypotension with percutaneous placement of a fibrin sealant". *Journal of Neurosurgery* **100**: 1098. doi:10.3171/jns.2004.100.6.1098.

[44]　Schievink, W. I. (2009). "A Novel Technique for Treatment of Intractable Spontaneous Intracranial Hypotension: Lumbar Dural Reduction Surgery". *Headache: the Journal of Head and Face Pain* **49** (7): 1047–1051. doi:10.1111/j.1526-4610.2009.01450.x. PMID 19473279.

[45]　Kitchel, SH; Eismont, FJ; Green, BA (1989). "Closed subarachnoid drainage for management of cerebrospinal fluid leakage after an operation on the spine". *The Journal of bone and joint surgery. American volume* **71** (7): 984–7. PMID 2760094.

[46]　Roosendaal, C. M.; Coppes, M. H.; Vroomen, P. C. A. J. (2009). "The paradox of intracranial hypotension responding well to CSF drainage". *European Journal of Neurology* **16** (12): e178. doi:10.1111/j.1468-1331.2009.02803.x. PMID 19863649.

[47]　Schwedt, TJ; Dodick, DW (2007). "Spontaneous intracranial hypotension". *Current pain and headache reports* **11** (1): 56–61. doi:10.1007/s11916-007-0023-9. PMID 17214923.

[48]　Schievink, W. I.; Maya, M. M.; Riedinger, M. (2003). "Recurrent spontaneous spinal cerebrospinal fluid leaks and intracranial hypotension: a prospective study". *Journal of Neurosurgery* **99**: 840. doi:10.3171/jns.2003.99.5.0840.

[49]　Mokri, B (2001). "Spontaneous intracranial hypotension". *Current pain and headache reports* **5** (3): 284–91. doi:10.1007/s11916-001-0045-7. PMID 11309218.

[50]　Stenzel, M.; Preuss, S.; Orloff, L.; Jecker, P.; Mann, W. (2005). "Cerebrospinal Fluid Leaks of Temporal Bone Origin: Etiology and Management". *ORL; journal for oto-rhino-laryngology and its related specialties* **67** (1): 51. doi:10.1159/000084306. PMID 15753623.

[51]　Schievink, W. I.; Maya, M. M. (2006). "Quadriplegia and cerebellar hemorrhage in spontaneous intracranial hypotension". *Neurology* **66** (11): 1777. doi:10.1212/01.wnl.0000218210.83855.40. PMID 16769965.

[52]　Alonso Cánovas, A; Martínez San Millán, J; Novillo López, ME; Masjuán Vallejo, J (2008). "Third cranial nerve palsy due to intracranial hypotension syndrome". *Neurologia (Barcelona, Spain)* **23** (7): 462–5. PMID 18726726.

[53]　Sayao, AL; Heran, MK; Chapman, K; Redekop, G; Foti, D (2009). "Intracranial hypotension causing reversible frontotemporal dementia and coma". *The Canadian journal of neurological sciences. Le journal canadien des sciences neurologiques* **36** (2): 252–6. PMID 19378725.

[54]　Ferrante, E.; Arpino, I.; Citterio, A.; Savino, A. (2009). "Coma resulting from spontaneous intracranial hypotension treated with the epidural blood patch in the Trendelenburg position pre-medicated with acetazolamide". *Clinical Neurology and Neurosurgery* **111** (8): 699. doi:10.1016/j.clineuro.2009.06.001. PMID 19577356.

[55]　Schievink, W. I.; Moser, F. G.; Pikul, B. K. (2007). "Reversal of coma with an injection of glue". *The Lancet* **369**: 1402. doi:10.1016/S0140-6736(07)60636-9.

[56]　Schievink, W. I.; Morreale, V. M.; Atkinson, J. L. D.; Meyer, F. B.; Piepgras, D. G.; Ebersold, M. J. (1998). "Surgical treatment of spontaneous spinal cerebrospinal fluid leaks". *Journal of Neurosurgery* **88** (2): 243–246. doi:10.3171/jns.1998.88.2.0243. PMID 9452231.

[57]　Ferrante, E.; Wetzl, R.; Savino, A.; Citterio, A.; Protti, A. (2004). "Spontaneous cerebrospinal fluid leak syndrome: report of 18 cases". *Neurological sciences : official journal of the Italian Neurological Society and of the Italian Society of Clinical Neurophysiology.* 25 **Suppl 3** (S3): S293–S295. doi:10.1007/s10072-004-0315-3. PMID 15549566.

[58]　Schievink, W.; Maya, M.; Pikul, B.; Louy, C. (2009). "Spontaneous spinal cerebrospinal fluid leaks as the cause of subdural hematomas in elderly patients on anticoagulation". *Journal of neurosurgery* **112** (2): 295–299. doi:10.3171/2008.10.JNS08428. PMID 19199465.

[59]　Larrosa, D; Vázquez, J; Mateo, I; Infante, J (2009). "Familial spontaneous intracranial hypotension". *Neurologia (Barcelona, Spain)* **24** (7): 485–7. PMID 19921558.

[60]　Schaltenbrand, G (1953). "Normal and pathological physiology of the cerebrospinal fluid circulation". *Lancet* **1** (6765): 805–8. doi:10.1016/S0140-6736(53)91948-5. PMID 13036182.

[61]　Mokri, B (2000). "Cerebrospinal fluid volume depletion and its emerging clinical/imaging syndromes". *Neurosurgical focus* **9** (1): e6. doi:10.3171/foc.2000.9.1.6. PMID 16859267.

[62]　Rupp, S. M.; Wilson, C. B. (1989). "Treatment of spontaneous cerebrospinal fluid leak with epidural blood patch". *Journal of Neurosurgery* **70** (5): 808. doi:10.3171/jns.1989.70.5.0808. PMID 2709124.

[63]　Carter, B.; Pasupuleti (2000). "Use of intravenous cosyntropin in the treatment of postdural puncture headache". *Anesthesiology* **92** (1): 272–274. doi:10.1097/00000542-200001000-00043. PMID 10638928.

[64]　Cánovas, L; Barros, C; Gómez, A; Castro, M; Castro, A (2002). "Use of intravenous tetracosactin in the treatment of postdural puncture headache: our experience in forty cases". *Anesthesia and analgesia* **94** (5): 1369. doi:10.1097/00000539-200205000-00069. PMID 11973227.

[65] Rouaud, T.; Lallement, F.; Choui, R.; Madigand, M. (2009). "Traitement de l'hypotension spontanée du liquide cérébrospinal par perfusion épidurale de sérum salé isotonique". *Revue Neurologique* **165** (2): 201. doi:10.1016/j.neurol.2008.05.006. PMID 19010507.

[66] Binder, DK; Dillon, WP; Fishman, RA; Schmidt, MH (2002). "Intrathecal saline infusion in the treatment of obtundation associated with spontaneous intracranial hypotension: technical case report". *Neurosurgery* **51** (3): 830–6; discussion 836–7. PMID 12188967.

[67] Schrijver, I.; Schievink, W. I.; Godfrey, M.; Meyer, F. B.; Francke, U. (2002). "Spontaneous spinal cerebrospinal fluid leaks and minor skeletal features of Marfan syndrome: a microfibrillopathy". *Journal of Neurosurgery* **96** (3): 483. doi:10.3171/jns.2002.96.3.0483. PMID 11883832.

Cerebrospinal fluid

Cerebrospinal fluid (CSF), *Liquor cerebrospinalis*, is a clear, colorless, bodily fluid, that occupies the subarachnoid space and the ventricular system around and inside the brain and spinal cord. In essence, the brain "floats" in it.

The CSF occupies the space between the arachnoid mater (the middle layer of the brain cover, meninges), and the pia mater (the layer of the meninges closest to the brain). It constitutes the content of all intra-cerebral (inside the brain, cerebrum) ventricles, cisterns, and sulci (singular sulcus), as well as the central canal of the spinal cord.

It acts as a "cushion" or buffer for the cortex, providing a basic mechanical and immunological protection to the brain inside the skull.

It is produced in the choroid plexus.

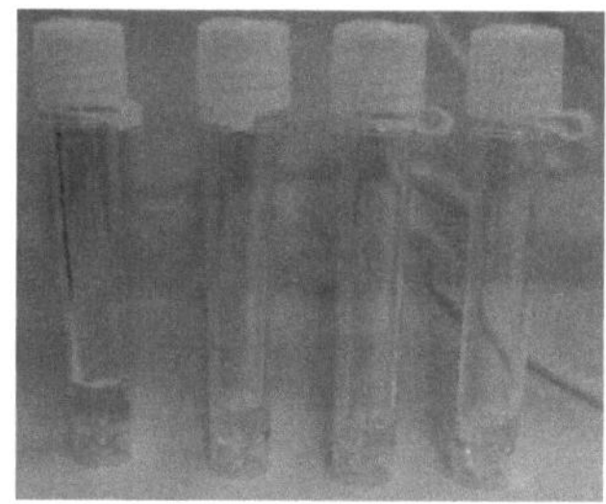

4 vials of CSF

Circulation

CSF is produced in the brain by modified ependymal cells in the choroid plexus (approx. 50-70%), and the remainder is formed around blood vessels and along ventricular walls. It circulates from the lateral ventricles to the foramen of Monro (Interventricular foramen), third ventricle, aqueduct of Sylvius (Cerebral aqueduct), fourth ventricle, foramen of Magendie (Median aperture) and foramina of Luschka (Lateral apertures); subarachnoid space over brain and spinal cord. CSF is reabsorbed into venous sinus blood via arachnoid granulations.

It had been thought that CSF returns to the vascular system by entering the dural venous sinuses via the arachnoid granulations (or villi). However, some[1] have suggested that CSF flow along the cranial nerves and spinal nerve roots allow it into the lymphatic channels; this flow may play a substantial role in CSF reabsorbtion, in particular in

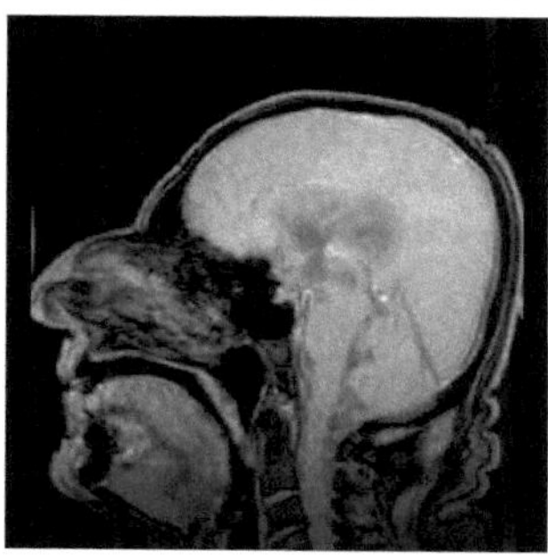

MRI showing pulsation of CSF

the neonate, in which arachnoid granulations are sparsely distributed. The flow of CSF to the nasal submucosal lymphatic channels through the cribriform plate seems to be especially important.[2]

Amount and constitution

The CSF is produced at a rate of 500 ml/day. Since the brain can contain only 135 to 150 ml, large amounts are drained primarily into the blood through arachnoid granulations in the superior sagittal sinus. Thus the CSF turns over about 3.7 times a day. This continuous flow into the venous system dilutes the concentration of larger, lipid-insoluble molecules penetrating the brain and CSF.[3]

The CSF contains approximately 0.3% plasma proteins, or approximately 15 to 40 mg/dL, depending on sampling site.[4]

CSF pressure, as measured by lumbar puncture (LP), is 10-18 cmH_2O (8-15 mmHg or 1.1-2 kPa) with the patient lying on the side and 20-30cmH_2O (16-24 mmHg or 2.1-3.2 kPa) with the patient sitting up.[5] In newborns, CSF pressure ranges from 8 to 10 cmH_2O (4.4–7.3 mmHg or 0.78–0.98 kPa). Most variations due to coughing or internal compression of jugular veins in the neck. When lying down, the cerebrospinal fluid as estimated by lumbar puncture is similar to the intracranial pressure.

There are quantitative differences in the distributions of a number of proteins in the CSF. In general, globular proteins and albumin are in lower concentration in ventricular CSF compared to lumbar or cisternal fluid.[6]

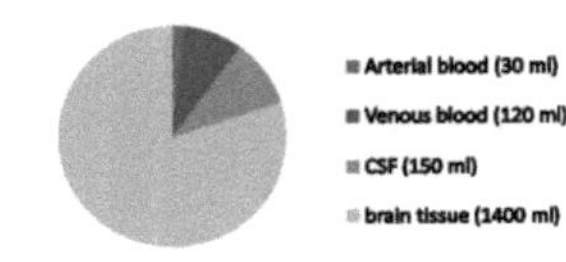

Intracranial volumetric distribution of cerebrospinal fluid, blood, and brain parenchyma

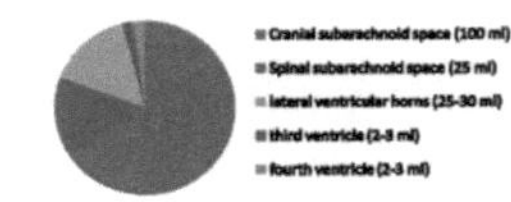

Volumetric distribution of cerebrospinal fluid

Reference ranges

Reference ranges for ions and metals in CSF

Substance	Lower limit	Upper limit	Unit	Corresponds to % of that in plasma
Osmolality	280[7]	300[7]	mmol/L	
Sodium	135[7]	150[7]	mmol/L	
Potassium	2.6[7]	3.0[7]	mmol/L	
Chloride	115[7]	130[7]	mmol/L	>100%[7]
Calcium	1.00[7]	1.40[7]	mmol/L	~50%[7]
Magnesium	1.2[7]	1.5[7]	mmol/L	>100%[7]
Iron	0.2[7]	0.4[7]	µmol/L	

Reference ranges for other molecules in CSF

Substance	Lower limit	Upper limit	Unit	Corresponds to % of that in plasma
Glucose	50[8]	80[8]	mg/dL	~60%[7]
	2.2,[9] 2.8[7]	3.9,[9] 4.4[7]	mmol/L	
Protein	15[7][8]	40,[4] 45[7][8]	mg/dL	~1%[7]
Lactate	1.1[7]	2.4[7]	mmol/L	
Creatinine	50[7]	110[7]	μmol/L	
Phosphorus	0.4[7]	0.6[7]	μmol/L	
Urea	3.0[7]	6.5[7]	mmol/L	
Carbon dioxide	20[7]	25[7]	mmol/L	

Reference ranges for other CSF constituents

Substance	Lower limit	Upper limit	Unit	Corresponds to % of that in blood plasma
RBCs	n/a[8]	0[8] / negative	cells/μL or cells/mm^3	
WBCs	0[8]	3[8]	cells/μL cells/mm^3	
pH	7.28[7]	7.32[7]	(unitless)	
PCO$_2$	44[7]	50[7]	mmHg	
	5.9[10]	6.7[10]	kPa	
PO$_2$	40[7]	44[7]	mmHg	
	5.3[10]	5.9[10]	kPa	

Functions

CSF serves four primary purposes:

1. Buoyancy: The actual mass of the human brain is about 1400 grams; however, the net weight of the brain suspended in the CSF is equivalent to a mass of 25 grams.[11] The brain therefore exists in neutral buoyancy, which allows the brain to maintain its density without being impaired by its own weight, which would cut off blood supply and kill neurons in the lower sections without CSF.[12]
2. Protection: CSF protects the brain tissue from injury when jolted or hit. In certain situations such as auto accidents or sports injuries, the CSF cannot protect the brain from forced contact with the skull case, causing hemorrhaging, brain damage, and sometimes death.[12]
3. Chemical stability: CSF flows throughout the inner ventricular system in the brain and is absorbed back into the bloodstream, rinsing the metabolic waste from the central nervous system through the blood-brain barrier. This allows for homeostatic regulation of the distribution of neuroendocrine factors, to which slight changes can cause problems or damage to the nervous system. For example, high glycine concentration disrupts temperature and blood pressure control, and high CSF pH causes dizziness and syncope.[12]

4. Prevention of brain ischemia: The prevention of brain ischemia is made by decreasing the amount of CSF in the limited space inside the skull. This decreases total intracranial pressure and facilitates blood perfusion.

Pathology and laboratory diagnosis

When CSF pressure is elevated, cerebral blood flow may be constricted. When disorders of CSF flow occur, they may therefore affect not only CSF movement but also craniospinal compliance and the intracranial blood flow, with subsequent neuronal and glial vulnerabilities. The venous system is also important in this equation. Infants and patients shunted as small children may have particularly unexpected relationships between pressure and ventricular size, possibly due in part to venous pressure dynamics. This may have significant treatment implications, but the underlying pathophysiology needs to be further explored.

CSF connections with the lymphatic system have been demonstrated in several mammalian systems. Preliminary data suggest that these CSF-lymph connections form around the time that the CSF secretory capacity of the choroid plexus is developing (in utero). There may be some relationship between CSF disorders, including hydrocephalus and impaired CSF lymphatic transport.

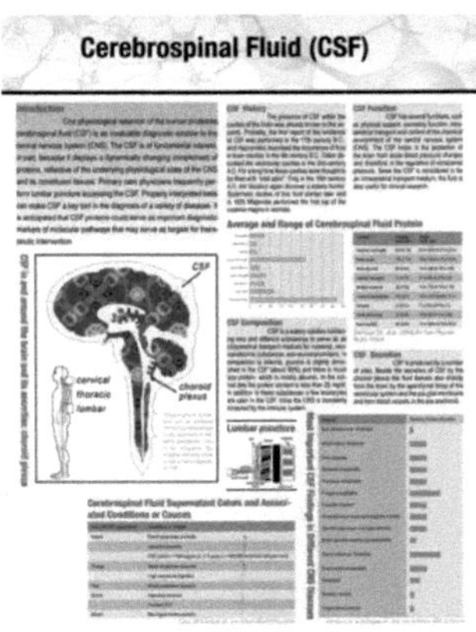
Cerebrospinal fluid (CSF) at glance.

CSF can be tested for the diagnosis of a variety of neurological diseases.[13] It is usually obtained by a procedure called lumbar puncture. Removal of CSF during lumbar puncture can cause a severe headache after the fluid is removed, because the brain hangs on the vessels and nerve roots, and traction on them stimulates pain fibers. The pain can be relieved by intrathecal injection of sterile isotonic saline. Lumbar puncture is performed in an attempt to count the cells in the fluid and to detect the levels of protein and glucose. These parameters alone may be extremely beneficial in the diagnosis of subarachnoid hemorrhage and central nervous system infections (such as meningitis). Moreover, a CSF culture examination may yield the microorganism that has caused the infection. By using more sophisticated methods, such as the detection of the oligoclonal bands, an ongoing inflammatory condition (for example, multiple sclerosis) can be recognized. A beta-2 transferrin assay is highly specific and sensitive for the detection for, e.g., CSF leakage.

Cause	Appearance	Polymorphonuclear cell	Lymphocyte	Protein	Glucose
Pyogenic bacterial meningitis	Yellowish, turbid	Markedly increased	Slightly increased or Normal	Markedly increased	Decreased
Viral meningitis	Clear fluid	Slightly increased or Normal	Markedly increased	Slightly increased or Normal	Normal
Tuberculous meningitis	Yellowish and viscous	Slightly increased or Normal	Markedly increased	Increased	Decreased
Fungal meningitis	Yellowish and viscous	Slightly increased or Normal	Markedly increased	Slightly increased or Normal	Normal or decreased

Lumbar puncture

Lumbar puncture can also be performed to measure the intracranial pressure, which might be increased in certain types of hydrocephalus. However a lumbar puncture should never be performed if increased intracranial pressure is suspected because it could lead to brain herniation and ultimately death.

Baricity

This fluid has an importance in anesthesiology. Baricity refers to the density of a substance compared to the density of human cerebral spinal fluid. Baricity is used in anesthesia to determine the manner in which a particular drug will spread in the intrathecal space.

Alzheimer's disease

A 2010 study showed analysis of CSF for three protein biomarkers can indicate the presence of Alzheimer's disease. The three biomarkers are CSF amyloid beta 1-42, total CSF tau protein and $P\text{-Tau}_{181P}$. In the study, the biomarker test showed good sensitivity, identifying 90% of persons with Alzheimer's disease, but poor specificity, as 36% of control subjects were positive for the biomarkers. The researchers suggested the low specificity may be explained by developing but not yet symptomatic disease in controls.[14] [15]

See also

- Meningitis
- CSF rhinorrhea
- Lumbar puncture
- Hydrocephalus
- Craniosacral therapy

References

[1] Zakharov A, Papaiconomou C, Djenic J, Midha R, Johnston M (2003). "Lymphatic CSF absorption pathways in neonatal sheep revealed by sub arachnoid injection of Microfil". *Neuropathol. Appl. Neurobiol.* **29** (6): 563–73. doi:10.1046/j.0305-1846.2003.00508.x. PMID 14636163.

[2] Johnston M (2003). "The importance of lymphatics in cerebrospinal fluid transport". *Lymphat. Res. Biol.* **1** (1): 41–4. doi:10.1089/15396850360495682. PMID 15624320.

[3] Saunders NR, Habgood MD, Dziegielewska KM (1999). "Barrier mechanisms in the brain, I. Adult brain". *Clin. Exp. Pharmacol. Physiol.* **26** (1): 11–9. doi:10.1046/j.1440-1681.1999.02986.x. PMID 10027064.

[4] Felgenhauer K (1974). "Protein size and CSF composition". *Klin. Wochenschr.* **52** (24): 1158–64. doi:10.1007/BF01466734. PMID 4456012.

[5] THE NORMAL CSF (http://neuropathology-web.org/chapter14/chapter14CSF.html) from Chapter Fourteen - Cerebrospinal Fluid. Neuropathology. By Dimitri Agamanolis, Northeast Ohio Medical University . Updated: May, 2011

[6] Merril CR, Goldman D, Sedman SA, Ebert MH (March 1981). "Ultrasensitive stain for proteins in polyacrylamide gels shows regional variation in cerebrospinal fluid proteins". *Science* **211** (4489): 1437–8. doi:10.1126/science.6162199. PMID 6162199.

[7] PATHOLOGY 425 CEREBROSPINAL FLUID [CSF] (http://www.pathology.ubc.ca/path425/SystemicPathology/Neuropathology/CerebrospinalFluidCSFDrGPBondy.rtf) at the Department of Pathology and Laboratory Medicine at the University of British Columbia. By Dr. G.P. Bondy. Retrieved November 2011

[8] Normal Reference Range Table (http://pathcuric1.swmed.edu/PathDemo/nrrt.htm) from The University of Texas Southwestern Medical Center at Dallas. Used in Interactive Case Study Companion to Pathologic basis of disease.

[9] Department of Chemical Pathology at the Chinese University of Hong Kong (http://www.cpy.cuhk.edu.hk/wardmanual/Menu/DP/Glucose.htm), in turn citing: Roberts WL et al. Reference Information for the Clinical Laboratory. In Tietz Textbook of Clinical Chemistry and Molecular Diagnostics, 4th edn. Burtis CA, Ashwood ER and Bruns DE eds. Elsevier Saunders 2006; 2251 - 2318

[10] Derived from mmHg values using 0.133322 kPa/mmHg

[11] Noback, Charles; Norman L. Strominger, Robert J. Demarest, David A. Ruggiero (2005). *The Human Nervous System.* Humana Press. p. 93. ISBN 978-1588290403.

[12] Saladin, Kenneth (2007). *Anatomy and Physiology: The Unity of Form and Function.* McGraw Hill. p. 520. ISBN 978-0-07-287506-5.,

[13] Seehusen DA, Reeves MM, Fomin DA (September 2003). "CSF analysis" (http://www.aafp.org/afp/20030915/1103.html). *Am Fam Physician* **68** (6): 1103–8. PMID 14524396. .

[14] De Meyer, Geert et al. (August 2010). "Diagnosis-Independent Alzheimer Disease Biomarker Signature in Cognitively Normal Elderly People" (http://archneur.ama-assn.org/cgi/content/short/67/8/949). *Archive of Neurology* **67** (8): 949–56. doi:10.1001/archneurol.2010.179. PMC 2963067. PMID 20697045. . Retrieved 2010-09-08.

[15] Herskovits, A. Zara; Growdon, John H. (August 2010). "Sharpen That Needle (editorial)" (http://archneur.ama-assn.org/cgi/content/extract/67/8/918). *Archive of Neurology* **67** (8): 918–20. doi:10.1001/archneurol.2010.151. PMID 20697041. . Retrieved 2010-09-08.

External links

- Circulation of Cerebrospinal Fluid (CSF) (http://www.aboutkidshealth.ca/En/HowTheBodyWorks/IntroductiontotheBrain/WhatisCerebrospinalFluidCSF/Pages/CirculationofCerebrospinalFluidCSF.aspx) - Interactive Tool

Dura mater

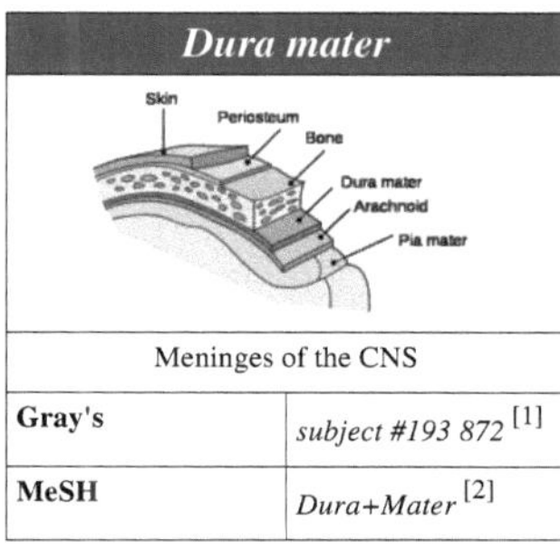

Meninges of the CNS	
Gray's	*subject #193 872* [1]
MeSH	*Dura+Mater* [2]

The **dura mater** /ˈdjʊərə ˈmeɪtər/, or **dura**, is the outermost of the three layers of the meninges surrounding the brain and spinal cord. It is derived from Mesoderm. The other two meningeal layers are the pia mater and the arachnoid mater. The dura surrounds the brain and the spinal cord and is responsible for keeping in the cerebrospinal fluid. The name *dura mater* is derived from the Latin "hard mother" or "tough mother", [3] [4] and is also referred to by the term "pachymeninx" (plural "pachymeninges"). The dura has been described as "tough and inflexible" and "leather-like".[3]

Layers and functions

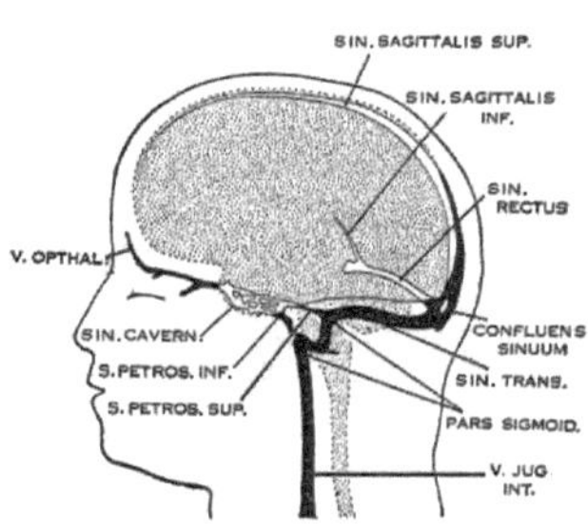

The dura mater has several functions and layers. The dura mater is a sac (aka thecal sac) that envelops the arachnoid mater. It surrounds and supports the dural sinuses (also called dural venous sinuses, cerebral sinuses, or cranial sinuses) and carries blood from the brain toward the heart.

The dura mater has two layers, or *lamellae*: The superficial layer, which serves as the skull's inner periosteum, called the endocranium; and a deep layer, the actual dura mater.

Dural folds and reflections

The dura separates into two layers at *dural reflections* (also known as *dural folds*), places where the inner dural layer is reflected as sheet-like protrusions into the cranial cavity. There are two main dural reflections:

- The tentorium cerebelli exists between and separates the cerebellum and brainstem from the occipital lobes of the cerebrum.[5]

- The falx cerebri, which separates the two hemispheres of the brain, is located in the longitudinal cerebral fissure between the hemispheres.[6]

Other two dural infoldings include the cerebellar falx and the sellar diaphragm

- The cerebellar falx (or **Falx cerebelli**) is a vertical dural infolding that lies inferior to the cerebellar tentorium in the posterior part of the posterior cranial fossa. It partially separates the cerebellar hemispheres.

- The sellar diaphragm is the smallest dural infolding and is a circular sheet of dura that is suspended between the clinoid processes, forming a partial roof over the hypophysial fossa. The sellar diaphgram covers the pituitary gland in this fossa and has an aperture for passage of the infundibulum (pituitary stalk) and hypophysial veins.

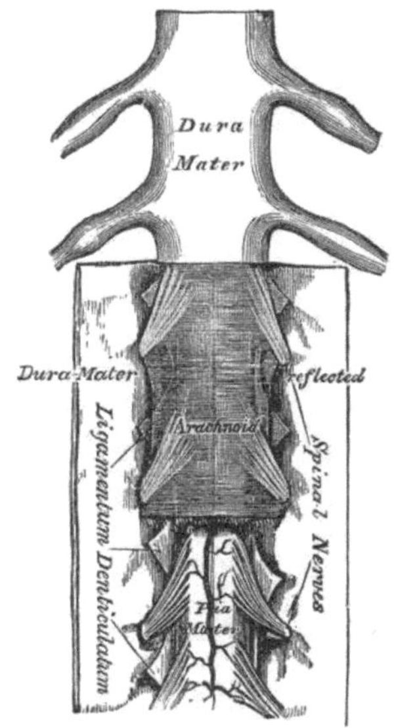

Spinal reflections and folds.

Drainage

The two layers of dura mater run together throughout most of the skull. Where they separate, the gap between them is called a dural venous sinus. These sinuses drain blood and cerebrospinal fluid from the brain and empty into the internal jugular vein.

They drain via the arachnoid villi, which are outgrowths of the arachnoid mater (the middle meningeal layer) that extend into the venous sinuses. These villi act as one-way valves.

Meningeal veins, which course through the dura mater, and **bridging veins**, which drain the underlying neural tissue and puncture the dura mater, empty into these dural sinuses. A rupture of a bridging vein causes a subdural hematoma.

Clinical significance

Many medical conditions involve the dura mater. A subdural hematoma occurs when there is an abnormal collection of blood between the dura and the arachnoid, usually as a result of torn bridging veins secondary to head trauma. An epidural hematoma is a collection of blood between the dura and the inner surface of the skull, and is usually due to arterial bleeding.

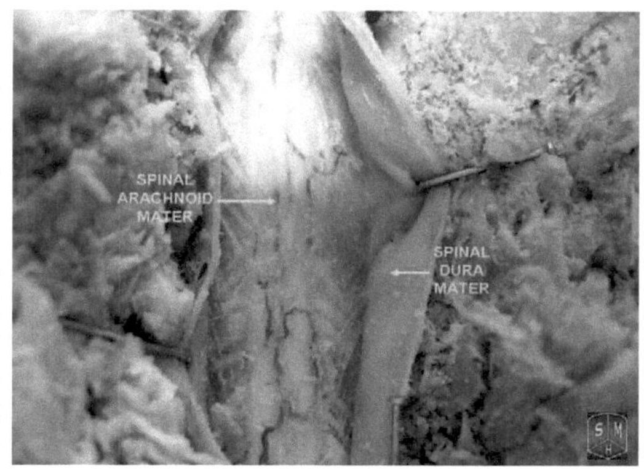

Spinal dura mater

In 2011, Scali et al., discovered a connection of soft tissue from the rectus capitis posterior major to the cervical dura mater. Various clinical manifestations may be linked to this anatomical relationship such as headaches, trigeminal neuralgia and other symptoms that involved the cervical dura (Spine 2011).[7] The rectus capitis posterior minor has a similar attachment as described by Hack et al. in 1995.

The dura-muscular, dura-ligamentous connections in the upper cervical spine and occipital areas may provide anatomic and physiologic answers to the cause of the cervicogenic headache. This proposal would further explain manipulation's efficacy in the treatment of cervicogenic headache.[8]

Blood supply

The middle meningeal artery supplies most of the blood for the dura mater, though the meningeal branches of the posterior and anterior ethmoidal artery also contribute.

Innervation

Sensory innervation of the supratentorial dura mater is via small meningeal branches of the trigeminal nerve (V1, V2 and V3).[9] The innervation for the infratentorial dura mater are upper cervical nerves.

The American Red Cross and some other agencies accepting blood donations consider dura mater transplants, along with receipt of pituitary-derived growth hormone, a risk factor due to concerns about Creutzfeldt-Jakob disease.[10]

Dural ectasia is the enlargement of the dura and is common in connective tissue disorders, such as Marfan Syndrome and Ehlers-Danlos Syndrome.

Spontaneous Cerebrospinal Fluid Leak is the fluid and pressure loss of spinal fluid due to holes in the dura mater.

References

[1]   http://education.yahoo.com/reference/gray/subjects/subject?id=193#p872

[2]   http://www.nlm.nih.gov/cgi/mesh/2011/MB_cgi?mode=&term=Dura+Mater

[3]   medterms.com (http://www.medterms.com/script/main/art.asp?articlekey=32512)

[4]   D. Harper - ety (http://www.etymonline.com/index.php?term=dura+mater)

[5]   Shepherd S. 2004. "Head Trauma." (http://www.emedicine.com/med/topic2820.htm) Emedicine.com.

[6]   Vinas FC and Pilitsis J. 2004. "Penetrating Head Trauma." (http://www.emedicine.com/med/topic2888.htm) Emedicine.com.

[7]   Frank Scali, Eric S. Marsili, Matt E. Pontell. "Anatomical Connection Between the Rectus Capitis Posterior Major and the Dura Mater" (http://journals.lww.com/spinejournal/Abstract/publishahead/Anatomical_Connection_Between_the_Rectus_Capitis.99006.aspx). *Spine.* .

[8]   Gary D. Hack, Peter Ratiu, John P. Kerr, Gwendolyn F. Dunn, Mi Young Toh. "Visualization of the Muscle-Dural Bridge in the Visible Human Female Data Set" (http://www.nlm.nih.gov/research/visible/vhp_conf/hack2/hack2.htm). *The Visible Human Project, National Library of Medicine.* .

[9]   'Gray's Anatomy for Students' 2005, Drake, Vogl and Mitchell, Elsevier

[10]   International Red Cross and Red Crescent Movement - redcross.org (http://www.redcross.org/services/biomed/0,1082,0_553_,00.html)

Additional images

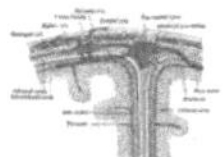

Diagrammatic representation of a section across the top of the skull, showing the membranes of the brain, etc.

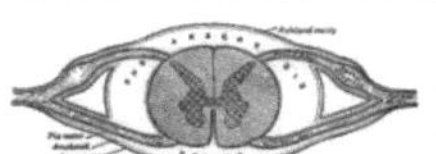

Diagrammatic transverse section of the medulla spinalis and its membranes.

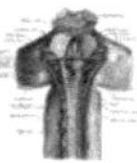

Upper part of medulla spinalis and hind- and mid-brains; posterior aspect, exposed in situ.

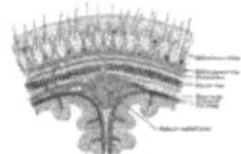

Diagrammatic section of scalp.

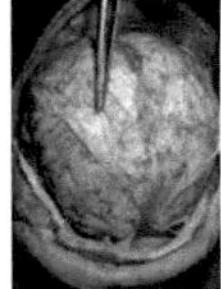

Autopsy photo from the CDC: The white "sheet" being held by the forceps is the dura mater.

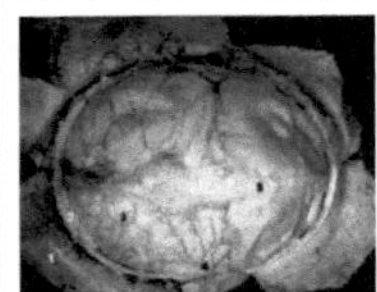

Human brain dura mater

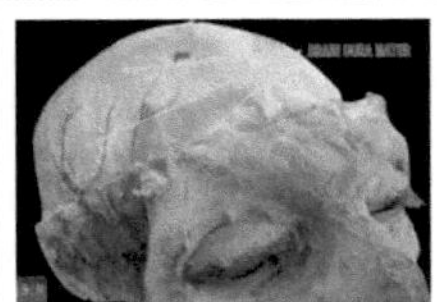

Dura mater

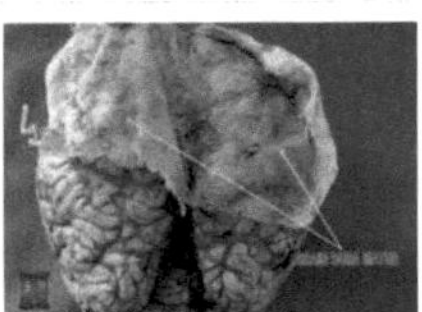

Cranian dura mater

External links

- *Dura+mater* (http://www.emedicinehealth.com/script/main/srchcont_dict.asp?src=Dura+mater) at eMedicine Dictionary

Meninges

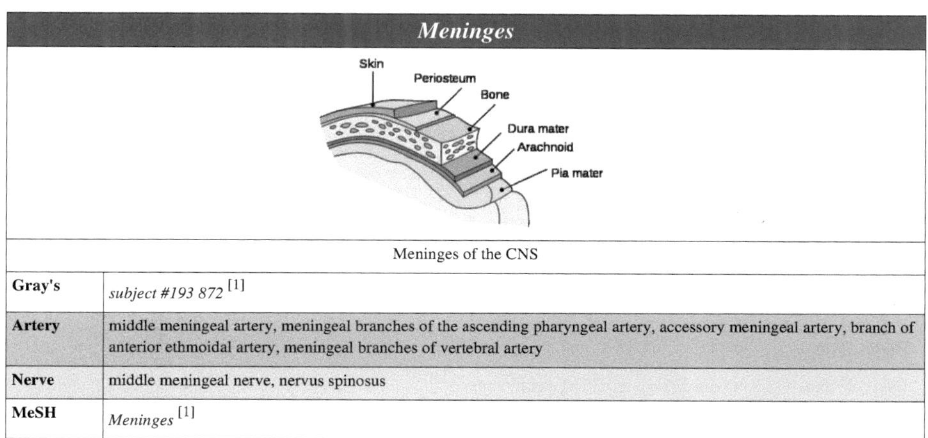

Meninges of the CNS	
Gray's	*subject #193 872* [1]
Artery	middle meningeal artery, meningeal branches of the ascending pharyngeal artery, accessory meningeal artery, branch of anterior ethmoidal artery, meningeal branches of vertebral artery
Nerve	middle meningeal nerve, nervus spinosus
MeSH	*Meninges* [1]

The **meninges** (singular **meninx** from the Greek μῆνιγξ, "membrane"[2]) is the system of membranes which envelopes the central nervous system. The meninges consist of three layers: the dura mater, the arachnoid mater, and the pia mater. The primary function of the meninges and of the cerebrospinal fluid is to protect the central nervous system.

Anatomy

Dura mater

The **dura mater** [Lt. Dura: Tough + mater: Mother](also rarely called meninx fibrosa, or pachymeninx) is a thick, durable membrane, closest to the skull. It consists of two layers, the periosteal layer which lies closest to the calvaria, and the inner meningeal layer which lies closer to the brain. It contains larger blood vessels which split into the capillaries in the pia mater. It is composed of dense fibrous tissue, and its inner surface is covered by flattened cells like those present on the surfaces of the pia mater and arachnoid. The dura mater is a sac which envelops the arachnoid and has been modified to serve several functions. The dura mater surrounds and supports the large venous channels (dural sinuses) carrying blood from the brain toward the heart.

Arachnoid mater

The middle element of the meninges is the **arachnoid mater**, so named because of its spider web-like appearance. It provides a cushioning effect for the central nervous system. The arachnoid mater exists as a thin, transparent membrane. It is composed of fibrous tissue and, like the pia mater, is covered by flat cells also thought to be impermeable to fluid. The arachnoid does not follow the convolutions of the surface of the brain and so looks like a loosely fitting sac. In the region of the brain, particularly, a large number of fine filaments called arachnoid trabeculae pass from the arachnoid through the subarachnoid space to blend with the tissue of the pia mater. The arachnoid and pia mater are sometimes together called the *leptomeninges.*

Pia mater

The pia or **pia mater**[Lt. Pia: Soft + mater: Mother] is a very delicate membrane. It is the meningeal envelope which firmly adheres to the surface of the brain and spinal cord. As such it follows all the minor contours of the brain (gyri and sulci). It is a very thin membrane composed of fibrous tissue covered on its outer surface by a sheet of flat cells thought to be impermeable to fluid. The pia mater is pierced by blood vessels which travel to the brain and spinal cord, and its capillaries are responsible for nourishing the brain.

Spaces

The subarachnoid space is the space which normally exists between the arachnoid and the pia mater, which is filled with cerebrospinal fluid.

Normally, the dura mater is attached to the skull, or to the bones of the vertebral canal in the spinal cord. The arachnoid is attached to the dura mater, while the pia mater is attached to the central nervous system tissue. When the dura mater and the arachnoid separate through injury or illness, the space between them is the subdural space.

Pathology

There are three types of hemorrhage involving the meninges:[3]

- A subarachnoid hemorrhage is acute bleeding under the arachnoid; it may occur spontaneously or as a result of trauma.
- A subdural hematoma is a hematoma (collection of blood) located in a separation of the arachnoid from the dura mater. The small veins which connect the dura mater and the arachnoid are torn, usually during an accident, and blood can leak into this area.
- An epidural hematoma similarly may arise after an accident or spontaneously.

Other medical conditions which affect the meninges include meningitis (usually from fungal, bacterial, or viral infection) and meningiomas arising from the meninges or from tumors formed elsewhere in the body which metastasize to the meninges.

Additional images

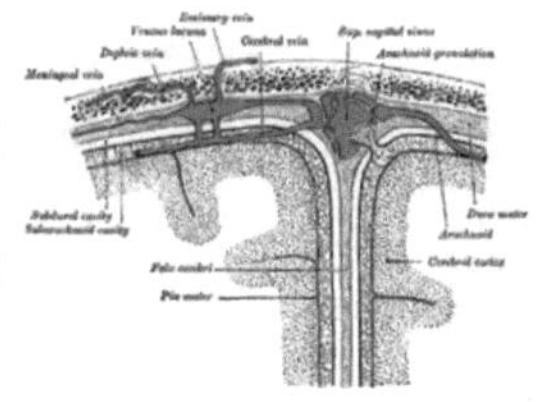

Diagrammatic representation of a section across the top of the skull

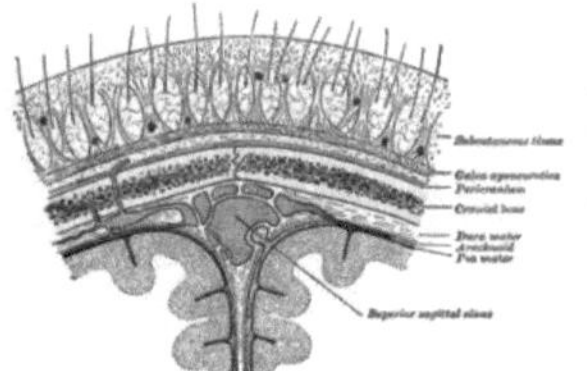

Diagrammatic section of scalp.

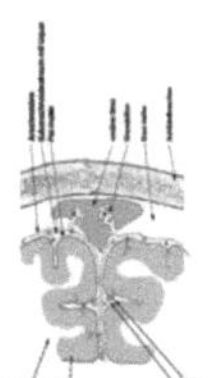

References

[1] http://www.nlm.nih.gov/cgi/mesh/2011/MB_cgi?mode=&term=Meninges

[2] μήνιγξ (http://www.perseus.tufts.edu/hopper/text?doc=Perseus:text:1999.04.0057:entry=mh=nigc), Henry George Liddell, Robert Scott, *A Greek-English Lexicon*, on Perseus

[3] Orlando Regional Healthcare, Education and Development. 2004. "Overview of Adult Traumatic Brain Injuries." (http://www. orlandoregional.org/pdf folder/overview adult brain injury.pdf) Retrieved on January 16, 2008.

Cerebrospinal fluid leak

A **cerebrospinal fluid leak** (**CSFL**) is a medical condition when the cerebrospinal fluid of a person leaks out of the dura mater.[1] [2] This can be caused by several reasons, including spontaneous cerebrospinal fluid leak, post-surgical lumbar puncture (iatrogenic), physical trauma, etc. While high CSF pressure can make reclining unbearable, low CSF pressure due to a leak is often relieved somewhat by maintaining a supine position.

References

[1] http://www.nlm.nih.gov/medlineplus/ency/article/001068.htm

[2] http://emedicine.medscape.com/article/338989-overview

Idiopathic

Idiopathic is an adjective used primarily in medicine meaning *arising spontaneously* or *from an obscure or unknown cause*. From Greek ἴδιος, idios (one's own) + πάθος, pathos (suffering), it means approximately "a disease of its own kind". It is technically a term from nosology, the classification of disease. For some medical conditions, one or more causes are somewhat understood, but in a certain percentage of people with the condition, the cause may not be readily apparent or characterized. In these cases, the origin of the condition is said to be idiopathic.

With some medical conditions, the medical community cannot establish a root cause for a large percentage of all cases (for example, focal segmental glomerulosclerosis or ankylosing spondylitis, the majority of which are idiopathic);[1] with other conditions, however, idiopathic cases account for a small percentage (for example, pulmonary fibrosis).[2] As medical and scientific advances are made with relation to a particular condition or disease, more root causes are discovered, and the percentage of cases designated as **idiopathic** decreases.

Popular references

In his book *The Human Body*, Isaac Asimov noted a comment about the term *idiopathic* made in the 20th edition of *Stedman's Medical Dictionary*: "*A high-flown term to conceal ignorance*".[3]

In the American television show *House*, the title character remarks that the word is "*from the Latin, meaning: 'We're idiots 'cause we can't figure out what's causing it.' "*[4]

See also

- Cryptogenic disease
- Diagnosis of exclusion
- Idiosyncratic drug reaction

References

[1] Daskalakis N, Winn M (2006). "Focal and segmental glomerulosclerosis". *Cell Mol Life Sci* **63** (21): 2506–11. doi:10.1007/s00018-006-6171-y. PMID 16952054.

[2] "Medical Encyclopedia: Idiopathic pulmonary fibrosis" (http://www.nlm.nih.gov/medlineplus/ency/article/000069.htm). *MedlinePlus*. . Retrieved 2007-02-13.

[3] Asimov, Isaac (1963). *The Human Body: Its Structure and Operation*. (http://books.google.com/?id=wn0hAAAAMAAJ&q=asimov+A+high-flown+term+to&dq=asimov+A+high-flown+term+to). Houghton Mifflin. pp. 179. ISBN 0-395-07350-2. .

[4] "http://www.twiztv.com/scripts/house/season1/house-117.htm"

Facial weakness

ICD-9	781.94 [1], 438.83 [2]

Facial weakness is a medical sign associated with a variety of medical conditions.

Some specific conditions associated with facial weakness include:

- stroke
- neurofibromatosis
- Bell's palsy
- Ramsay Hunt syndrome
- Spontaneous cerebrospinal fluid leak

See also

- Acute facial nerve paralysis
- Facioscapulohumeral muscular dystrophy

External links

- Differential diagnosis [3]
- Diagram of appearance in stroke [4]

References

[1] http://www.icd9data.com/getICD9Code.ashx?icd9=781.94
[2] http://www.icd9data.com/getICD9Code.ashx?icd9=438.83
[3] http://pediatricneuro.com/alfonso/pg169.htm
[4] http://www.littletongov.org/fire/ems/hot/2004/stroke/facialweakenss.jpg

Epidural blood patch

An **epidural blood patch** is a surgical procedure which uses autologous blood in order to close one or many holes in the dura mater of the spinal cord, usually as a result of a previous lumbar puncture. The procedure can be used to relieve post dural puncture headaches caused by lumbar puncture (spinal tap). A small amount of the patient's blood is injected into the epidural space near the site of the original puncture; the resulting blood clot then "patches" the meningeal leak. The procedure carries the typical risks of any epidural puncture. However, it is effective,[1] and further intervention is rarely necessary.

An epidural needle is inserted into the epidural space at the site of the cerebrospinal fluid leak and blood is injected. The clotting factors of the blood close the hole in the dura.

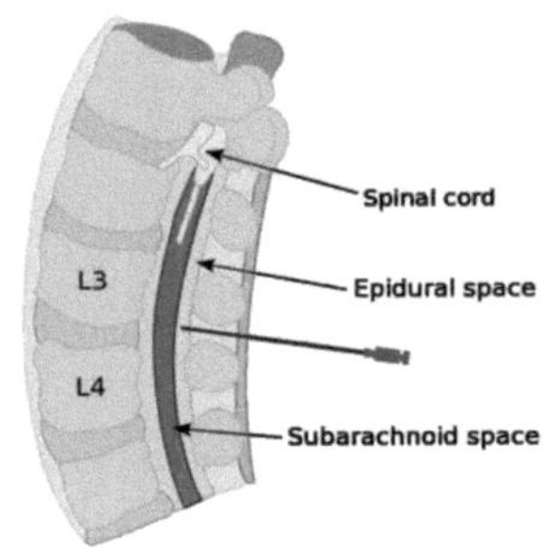

Epidural blood patch.

As such, the autologous blood does not "repair" the leak, but rather treats the patient's symptomology.

It is also postulated that the relief of the headache after an epidural blood patch is due to more of a compression effect than sealing the leak. Because the fluid column in the lumbar spine is continuous with the fluid around the brain, the blood exerts a "squeeze" and relieves the low pressure state in the head.

References

[1] Safa-Tisseront V, Thormann F, Malassiné P, *et al.* (August 2001). "Effectiveness of epidural blood patch in the management of post-dural puncture headache" (http://meta.wkhealth.com/pt/pt-core/template-journal/lwwgateway/media/landingpage.htm?issn=0003-3022& volume=95&issue=2&spage=334). *Anesthesiology* **95** (2): 334–9. PMID 11506102. .

Taken from http:/ / www. uwhealth. org/ servlet/ Satellite?cid=1105110029981& pagename=B_EXTRANET_HEALTH_INFORMATION/FlexMember/Show_Public_HFFY&c=FlexGroup

Georg Schaltenbrand

Georg Schaltenbrand	
Georg Schaltenbrand	
Born	26 November 1897Oberhausen
Died	24 October 1979 (aged 81)Würzburg
Nationality	German
Fields	neurologist

Georg Schaltenbrand (26 November 1897–24 October 1979) was a German neurologist known for his work on Cerebrospinal fluid.

References

- Collmann, Hartmut (2008). "Georges Schaltenbrand (26. 11. 1897 24. 10. 1979)". *Würzburger medizinhistorische Mitteilungen / im Auftrage der Würzburger medizinhistorischen Gesellschaft und in Verbindung mit dem Institut für Geschichte der Medizin der Universität Würzburg* (Germany) **27**: 63–92. ISSN 0177-5227. PMID 19230367.
- Hopf, H C (1980). "Georges Schaltenbrand (1897-1979)". *J. Neurol.* (GERMANY, WEST) **223** (3): 153–8. ISSN 0340-5354. PMID 6157008.

Spinal canal

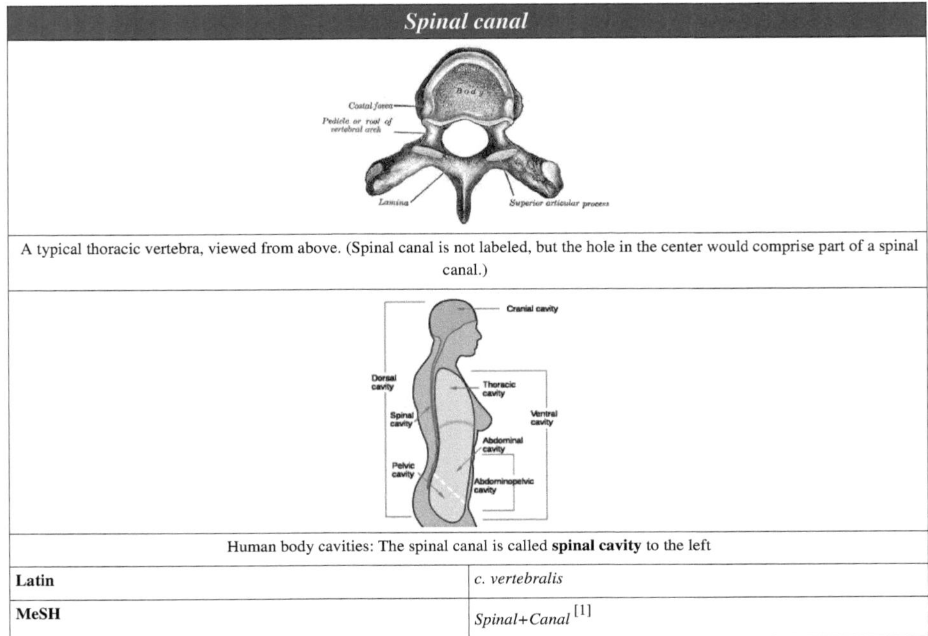

A typical thoracic vertebra, viewed from above. (Spinal canal is not labeled, but the hole in the center would comprise part of a spinal canal.)

Human body cavities: The spinal canal is called **spinal cavity** to the left

Latin	c. vertebralis
MeSH	Spinal+Canal [1]

The **spinal canal** (or **vertebral canal** or **spinal cavity**) is the space in vertebrae through which the spinal cord passes. It is a process of the dorsal human body cavity. This canal is enclosed within the vertebral foramen of the vertebrae. In the intervertebral spaces, the canal is protected by the ligamentum flavum posteriorly and the posterior longitudinal ligament anteriorly.

The outermost layer of the meninges, the dura mater, is closely associated with the arachnoid which in turn is loosely connected to the innermost layer of the meninges, the pia mater. The meninges divide the spinal canal into the epidural space and the subarachnoid space. The pia mater is closely attached to the spinal cord. A subdural space is generally only present due to trauma and/or pathological situations. The subarachnoid space is filled with cerebrospinal fluid and contains the vessels that supply the spinal cord, namely the anterior spinal artery and the paired posterior spinal arteries, accompanied by a corresponding spinal veins. The spinal arteries form anastomoses known as the vasocorona of the spinal cord. The epidural space contains loose fatty tissue, and a network of large, thin-walled blood vessels called the internal vertebral venous plexuses.

The spinal canal was first described by Jean Fernel.

External links

- Diagram at wisc.edu [2]

References

[1] http://www.nlm.nih.gov/cgi/mesh/2011/MB_cgi?mode=&term=Spinal+Canal
[2] http://www.orthorehab.wisc.edu/rehab/interventionalpainprogram/images/spinal_Canalnew2.jpg

Orthostatic headache

Orthostatic headache is a medical condition in which a person develops a severe headache while vertical and the headache is relieved when horizontal.[1] [2] [3]

Causes

There exist many reasons for orthostatic headaches. One reason is a spontaneous cerebrospinal fluid leak.

References

[1] http://www.neurology.org/cgi/content/abstract/71/23/1902
[2] http://findarticles.com/p/articles/mi_hb4365/is_/ai_n29235360
[3] http://www3.interscience.wiley.com/journal/118976414/abstract

Dysgeusia

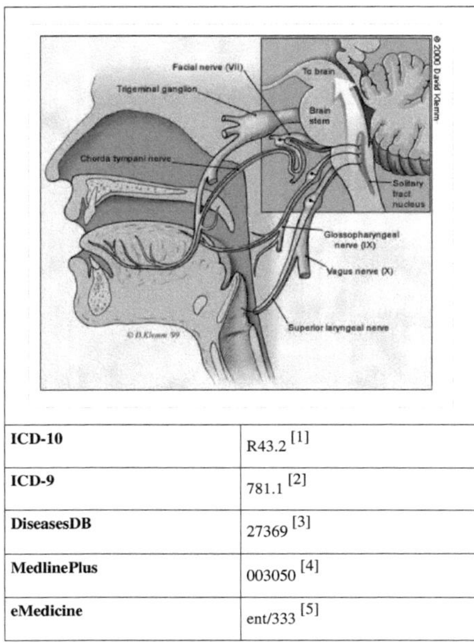

ICD-10	R43.2 [1]
ICD-9	781.1 [2]
DiseasesDB	27369 [3]
MedlinePlus	003050 [4]
eMedicine	ent/333 [5]

Dysgeusia (/dɪsˈgjuːziə/ *dis-gew-zee-ə*) is the distortion of the sense of taste. Dysgeusia is also often associated with ageusia, which is the complete lack of taste, and hypogeusia, which is the decrease in taste sensitivity.[6] An alteration in taste or smell may be a secondary process in various disease states, or it may be the primary symptom. The distortion in the sense of taste is the only symptom, and diagnosis is usually complicated since the sense of taste is tied together with other sensory systems. Common causes of dysgeusia include chemotheraphy, asthma treatment with albuterol, and zinc deficiency. Different drugs could also be responsible for altering taste and resulting in dysgeusia. Due to the variety of causes of dysgeusia, there are many possible treatments that are effective in alleviating or terminating the symptoms of dysgeusia. These include artificial saliva, pilocarpine, zinc supplementation, alterations in drug therapy, and alpha lipoic acid.

Background

The sense of taste is based on the detection of chemicals by specialized taste cells in the mouth. The mouth, throat, larynx, and esophagus all have taste buds, which are replaced every ten days. Each taste bud contains receptor cells.[7] Afferent nerves make contact with the receptor cells at the base of the taste bud.[8] A single taste bud is innervated by several afferent nerves, while a single efferent fiber innervates several taste buds.[9] Fungiform papillae are present on the anterior portion of the tongue while circumvallate papillae and foliate papillae are found on the posterior portion of the tongue. The salivary glands are responsible for keeping the taste buds moist with saliva.[10]

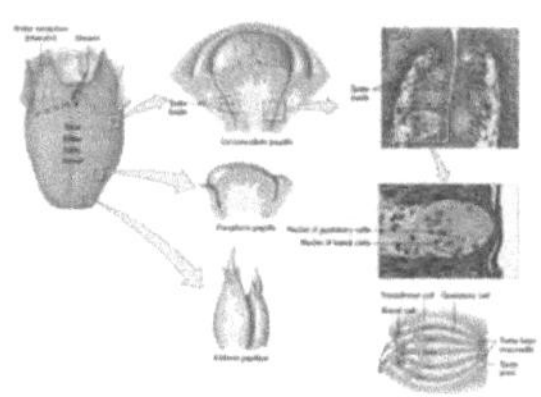

Taste Receptors of the Tongue.

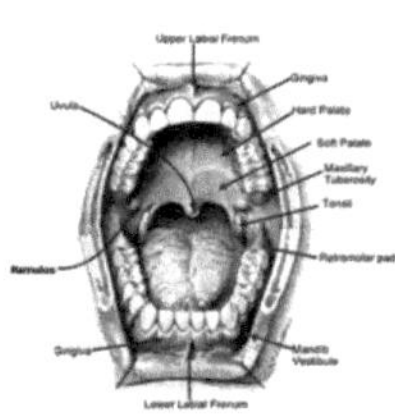

The Oral Cavity.

A single taste bud is composed of four different types of cells, and each taste bud has at least 30 to 80 cells. Type I cells are thinly shaped, usually in the periphery of other cells. They also contain high amounts of chromatin. Type II cells have prominent nuclei and nucleoli with much less chromatin than Type I cells. Type III cells have multiple mitochondria and large vesicles. Type I, II, and III cells also contain synapses. Type IV cells are normally rooted at the posterior end of the taste bud. Every cell in the taste bud forms microvilli at the ends.[11]

In humans, the sense of taste is conveyed via three of the twelve cranial nerves. The facial nerve (VII) is responsible for taste sensations from the anterior two thirds of the tongue, the glossopharyngeal nerve (IX) is responsible for taste sensations from the posterior one third of the tongue while a branch of the vagus nerve (X) carries some taste sensations from the back of the oral cavity.

Symptoms

The alterations in the sense of taste, usually a metallic taste, and sometimes smell are the only symptoms.[12] The duration of the symptoms of dysgeusia depends on the cause. If the alteration in the sense of taste is due to gum disease, dental plaque, a temporary medication, or a short-term condition such as a cold, the dysgeusia should disappear once the cause is removed. In some cases, if lesions are present in the taste pathway and nerves have been damaged, the dysgeusia may be permanent.

Diagnosis

In general, gustatory disorders are challenging to diagnose and evaluate. Because gustatory functions are tied to the sense of smell, the somatosensory system, and the perception of pain (such as in tasting spicy foods), it is difficult to examine sensations mediated through an individual system.[13] In addition, gustatory dysfunction is rare when compared to olfactory disorders.[14]

Diagnosis of dysgeusia begins with the patient being questioned about salivation, swallowing, chewing, oral pain, previous ear infections (possibly indicated by hearing or balance problems), oral hygiene, and stomach problems.[15] The initial history assessment also considers the possibility of accompanying diseases such as diabetes mellitus, hypothyroidism, or cancer.[15] A clinical examination is conducted and includes an inspection of the tongue and the oral cavity. Furthermore, the ear canal is inspected, as lesions of the chorda tympani have a predilection for this site.[15]

Gustatory testing

In order to further classify the extent of dysgeusia and clinically measure the sense of taste, gustatory testing may be performed. Gustatory testing is performed either as a whole-mouth procedure or as a regional test. In both techniques, natural or electrical stimuli can be used. In regional testing, 20 to 50 µL of liquid stimulus is presented to the anterior and posterior tongue using a pipette, soaked filter-paper disks, or cotton swabs.[14] In whole mouth testing, small quantities (2-10 mL) of solution are administered, and the patient is asked to swish the solution around in the mouth.[14]

Threshold tests for sucrose (sweet), citric acid (sour), sodium chloride (salty), and quinine or caffeine (bitter) are frequently performed with natural stimuli. One of the most frequently used techniques is the "three-drop test."[16] In this test, three drops of liquid are presented to the subject. One of the drops is of the taste stimulus, and the other two drops are pure water.[16] Threshold is defined as the concentration at which the patient identifies the taste correctly three times in a row.[16]

Suprathreshold tests, which provide intensities of taste stimuli above threshold levels, are used to assess the patient's ability to differentiate between different intensities of taste and to estimate the magnitude of suprathreshold loss of taste. From these tests, ratings of pleasantness can be obtained using either the direct scaling or magnitude matching method and may be of value in the diagnosis of dysgeusia. Direct scaling tests show the ability to discriminate among different intensities of stimuli and whether a stimulus of one quality (sweet) is stronger or weaker than a stimulus of another quality (sour).[17] Direct scaling cannot be used to determine if a taste stimulus is being perceived at abnormal levels. In this case, magnitude matching is used, in which a patient is asked to rate the intensities of taste stimuli and stimuli of another sensory system, such as the loudness of a tone, on a similar scale.[17] For example, the Connecticut Chemosensory Clinical Research Center asks patients to rate the intensities of NaCl, sucrose, citric acid and quinine-HCl stimuli, and the loudness of 1000 Hz tones.[17] Assuming normal hearing, the results of this cross-sensory test show the relative strength of the sense of taste in relation to the loudness of the auditory stimulus. Although many of the tests are based on ratings using the direct scaling method, some tests do use the magnitude-matching procedure.

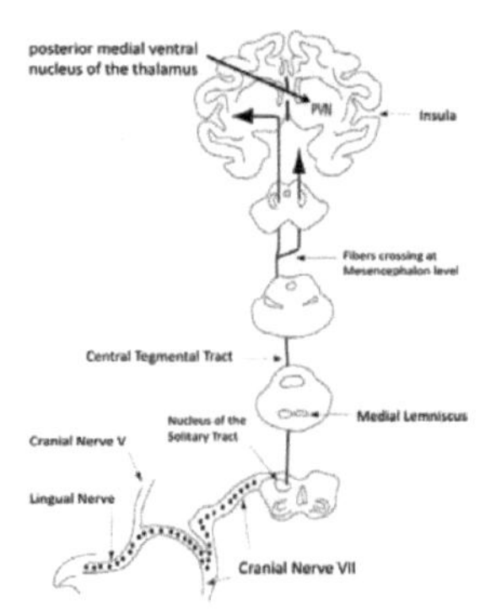

Schematic drawing of the current understanding of the Gustatory pathway.

Other tests include identification or discrimination of common taste substances. Topical anesthesia of the tongue has been reported to be of use in the diagnosis of dysgeusia as well, since it has been shown to relieve the symptoms of dysgeusia temporarily.[14] In addition to techniques based on the administration of chemicals to the tongue, electrogustometry is frequently used. It is based on the induction of gustatory sensations by means of an anodal electrical direct current. Patients usually report sour or metallic sensations similar to those associated with touching both poles of a live battery to the tongue.[18] Although electrogustometry is widely used, there seems to be a poor correlation between electrically and chemically induced sensations.[19]

Diagnostic tools

Certain diagnostic tools can also be used to help determine the extent of dysgeusia. Electrophysiological tests and simple reflex tests may be applied to identify abnormalities in the nerve-to-brainstem pathways. For example, the blink reflex may be used to evaluate the integrity of the trigeminal nerve–pontine brainstem–facial nerve pathway, which may play a role in gustatory function.[20]

Structural imaging is routinely used to investigate lesions in the taste pathway. Magnetic resonance imaging allows direct visualization of the cranial nerves.[21] Furthermore, it provides significant information about the type and cause of a lesion.[21] Analysis of mucosal blood flow in the oral cavity in combination with the assessment of autonomous cardiovascular factors appears to be useful in the diagnosis of autonomic nervous system disorders in burning mouth syndrome and in patients with inborn disorders, both of which are associated with gustatory dysfunction.[22] Cell cultures may also be used when fungal or bacterial infections are suspected.

In addition, the analysis of saliva should be performed, as it constitutes the environment of taste receptors, including transport of tastes to the receptor and protection of the taste receptor.[23] Typical clinical investigations involve sialometry and sialochemistry.[23] Studies have shown that electron micrographs of taste receptors obtained from saliva samples indicate pathological changes in the taste buds of patients with dysgeusia and other gustatory disorders.[24]

Causes

Chemotherapy

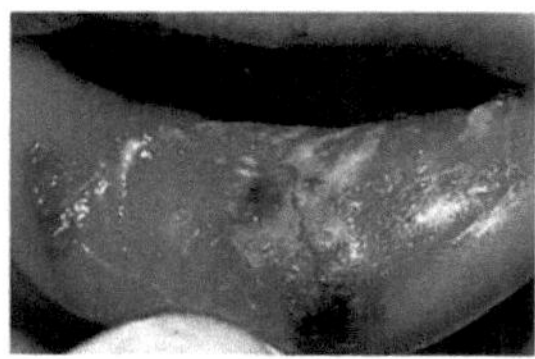

Oral Mucositis in a patient undergoing chemotherapy.

A major cause of dysgeusia is antineoplastic chemotherapy. Chemotherapy often induces damage to the oral cavity, resulting in oral mucositis, oral infection, and salivary gland dysfunction. Oral mucositis consists of inflammation of the mouth, along with sores and ulcers in the tissues.[25] Healthy individuals normally have a diverse range of microbial organisms residing in their oral cavities; however, chemotherapy can permit these typically non-pathogenic agents to cause serious infection, which may result in a decrease in saliva. In addition, patients who undergo radiation therapy also lose salivary tissues.[26] Saliva is an important component of the taste mechanism. Saliva both interacts with and protects the taste receptors in the mouth.[27] Saliva mediates sour and sweet tastes through bicarbonate ions and glutamate, respectively.[28] The salt taste is induced when sodium chloride levels surpass the concentration in the saliva.[28] It has been reported that 50% of chemotherapy patients have suffered from either dysgeusia or another form of taste impairment.[25] Examples of chemotherapy treatments that can lead to dysgeusia are cyclophosphamide, cisplatin, and etoposide.[25] The exact mechanism of chemotherapy-induced dysgeusia is unknown.[25]

Taste buds

Distortions in the taste buds may give rise to dysgeusia. In one study conducted by Masahide Yasuda and Hitoshi Tomita from Nihon University of Japan, it has been observed that patients suffering from this taste disorder have less microvilli than normal. In addition, the nucleus and cytoplasm of the taste bud cells have been reduced. Based on their findings, dygeusia results from loss of microvilli and the reduction of Type III intracellular vesicles, all of which could potentially interfere with the gustatory pathway.[11]

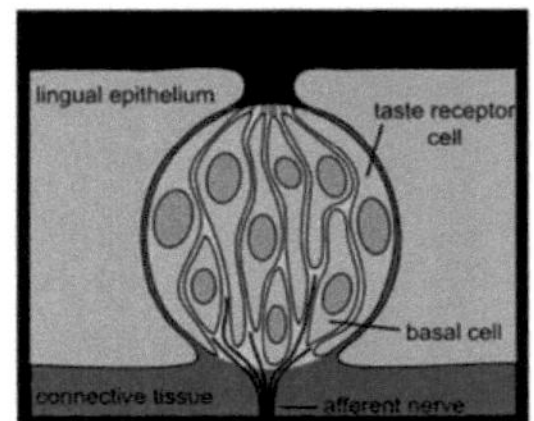

The anatomy of the taste bud.

Zinc deficiency

■ Table 10-6. Drugs That May Cause Taste Disorders	
Drug Category	**Examples**
Antihelminthic	Levamisole
Antithyroid	Carbimazole, methylthiouracil, propylthiouracil
Antiseptic	Chlorhexidine
Anti-inflammatory	Penicillamine, colchicine, gold salts, allopurinol, nonsteroidal anti-inflammatory drugs
Antimitotic	Bleomycin, α-interferon, interleukin-2, methotrexate, vincristine, doxorubicin, chlorambucil, procarbazine, cisplatin, 5-fluorouracil
Antifungal	Amphotericin B, griseofulvin
Antibiotic	Tetracycline, sulfonamides, penicillins, cephalosporins, ethambutol
Antiprotozoal	Metronidazole, pentamidine
Antiviral	Idoxuridine, zidovudine, didanosine, protease inhibitors (e.g., indinavir, ritonavir)
Calcium channel blocker	Nifedipine, amlodipine, diltiazem
Anticholinergic	Benzhexol, tricyclic antidepressants, oxybutynin
Diuretic	Acetazolamide, amiloride, frusemide, hydrochlorothiazide
Antiarrhythmic	Amiodarone, procainamide, propranolol
Oral hypoglycemic agents	Phenformin, glipizide
Antiepileptic	Phenytoin, carbamazepine
Antipsychotic or antidepressant	Trifluoperazine, lithium carbonate, amitriptyline, clomipramine, paroxetine, sertraline
Drugs used in Parkinson's disease	Levodopa, pergolide, benzhexol, selegiline
Miscellaneous	Theobromine, theophylline, quinine, strychnine, sumatriptan nasal spray, metoclopramide, cimetidine, disulfiram, pesticides, lead, industrial solvents and paints

Drugs Affecting Taste.

Another primary cause of dysgeusia is zinc deficiency. While the exact role of zinc in dysgeusia is unknown, it has been cited that zinc is partly responsible for the repair and production of taste buds. Zinc somehow directly or indirectly interacts with carbonic anhydrase VI, influencing the concentration of gustin, which is linked to the production of taste buds.[29] It has also been reported that patients treated with zinc experience an elevation in calcium concentration in the saliva.[29] In order to work properly, taste buds rely on calcium receptors.[30] Zinc "is an important cofactor for alkaline phosphatase, the most abundant enzyme in taste bud membranes; it is also a component of a parotid salivary protein important to the development and maintenance of normal taste buds."[30]

Drugs

There are also a wide variety of drugs that can trigger dysgeusia, including H1-antihistamines, such as azelastine and emedastine.[31] Approximately 250 drugs affect taste.[32] The sodium channels linked to taste receptors can be inhibited by amiloride, and the creation of new taste buds and saliva can be impeded by antiproliferative drugs.[32] Saliva can have traces of the drug, giving rise to a metallic flavor in the mouth; examples include lithium carbonate and tetracyclines.[32] Drugs containing sulfhydryl groups, including penicillamine and captopril, may react with zinc and cause deficiency.[30] Metronidazole and chlorhexidine have been found to interact with metal ions that associate with the cell membrane.[33] Drugs that prevent the production of angiotensin II by inhibiting angiotensin converting enzyme, eprosartan for example, have been linked to dysgeusia.[34]

Miscellaneous causes

Xerostomia, also known as dry mouth syndrome, can precipitate dysgeusia because normal salivary flow and concentration are necessary for taste. Injury to the glossopharyngeal nerve can result in dysgeusia. In addition, damage done to the pons, thalamus, and midbrain, all of which compose the gustatory pathway, can be potential factors.[35] In a case study, 22% of patients who were experiencing a bladder obstruction were also suffering from dysgeusia. Dysgeusia was eliminated in 100% of these patients once the obstruction was removed.[35] Although it is uncertain what the relationship between bladder relief and dysgeusia entails, it has been observed that the areas responsible for urinary system and taste in the pons and cerebral cortex in the brain are close in proximity.[35]

Many of the causes for dysgeusia are not fully understood, making idiopathic dysgeusia very common. A wide range of miscellaneous factors may contribute to this taste disorder, such as gastric reflux, lead poisoning, and diabetes mellitus.[7] A minority of pine nuts can apparently cause taste disturbances, for reasons which are not entirely proven. Certain pesticides can have damaging effects on the taste buds and nerves in the mouth. These pesticides include organochloride compounds and carbamate pesticides. Damage to the peripheral nerves, along with injury to the chorda tympani branch of the facial nerve, also cause dysgeusia.[7] A surgical risk for laryngoscopy and tonsillectomy include dysgeusia.[7] Patients who suffer from the burning mouth syndrome, most likely menopausal women, are often suffering from dysgeusia as well.[36]

Treatments

Artificial saliva and pilocarpine

Because medications have been linked to approximately 22% to 28% of all cases of dysgeusia, researching a treatment for this particular cause has been important.[37] Xerostomia, or a decrease in saliva flow, can be a side effect of many drugs, which, in turn, can lead to the development of taste disturbances such as dysgeusia.[37] Patients can lessen the effects of xerostomia with breath mints, sugarless gum, or lozenges, or physicians can increase saliva flow with artificial saliva or oral pilocarpine.[37] Artificial saliva mimics the characteristics of natural saliva by lubricating and protecting the mouth but does not provide any digestive or enzymatic benefits.[38] Pilocarpine is a cholinergic drug meaning it has the same effects as the neurotransmitter acetylcholine. Acetylcholine has the function of stimulating the salivary glands to actively produce saliva.[39] The increase in saliva flow is effective in improving the movement of tastants to the taste buds.[37]

Zinc deficiency

Zinc supplementation

Approximately one half of drug-related taste distortions are caused by a zinc deficiency.[37] Many medications are known to chelate, or bind, zinc preventing the element from functioning properly.[37] Due to the causal relationship of insufficient zinc levels to taste disorders, research has been conducted to test the efficacy of zinc supplementation as a possible treatment for dygeusia. In a randomized

Zinc Gluconate.

clinical trial, fifty patients suffering from idiopathic dysgeusia were given either zinc or a lactose placebo.[29] The patients prescribed the zinc reported experiencing improved taste function and less severe symptoms compared to the control group, suggesting that zinc may be a beneficial treatment.[29] The efficacy of zinc, however, has been ambiguous in the past. In a second study, 94% of patients who were provided with zinc supplementation did not experience any improvement in their condition.[37] This ambiguity is most likely due to small sample sizes and the wide range of causes of dysgeusia.[29] A recommended daily oral dose of 25–100 mg appears to be an effective treatment for taste dysfunction provided that there are low levels of zinc in the blood serum.[40] There is not a sufficient amount of evidence to determine whether or not zinc supplementation is able to treat dysgeusia when low zinc concentrations are not detected in the blood.[40]

Zinc infusion in chemotherapy

It has been reported that approximately 68% of cancer patients undergoing chemotherapy experience disturbances in sensory perception such as dysgeusia.[41] In a pilot study involving twelve lung cancer patients, chemotherapy drugs were infused with zinc in order to test its potential as a treatment.[42] The results indicated that, after two weeks, no taste disturbances were reported by the patients who received the zinc-supplemented treatment while most of the patients in the control group who did not receive the zinc reported taste alterations.[42] A multi-institutional study involving a larger sample size of 169 patients, however, indicated that zinc-infused chemotherapy did not have an effect on the development of taste disorders in cancer patients.[41] An excess amount of zinc in the body can have negative effects on the immune system, and physicians must use caution when administering zinc to immunocompromised cancer patients.[41] Because taste disorders can have detrimental effects on a patient's quality of life, more research needs to be conducted concerning possible treatments such as zinc supplementation.[43]

Altering drug therapy

The effects of drug-related dysgeusia can oftentimes be reversed by stopping the patient's regimen of the taste altering medication.[44] In one case, a forty-eight-year-old woman who was suffering from hypertension was being treated with valsartan.[45] Due to this drug's inability to treat her condition, she began taking a regimen of eprosartan, an angiotensin II receptor antagonist.[45] Within three weeks, she began experiencing a metallic taste and a burning sensation in her mouth that ceased when she stopped taking the medication.[45] When she began taking eprosartan on a second occasion, her dysgeusia returned.[45] In a second case, a fifty-nine-year-old man was prescribed amlodipine in order to treat his hypertension.[46] After eight years of taking the drug, he developed a loss of taste sensation and numbness in his tongue.[46] When he ran out of his medication, he decided not to obtain a refill and stopped taking amlodipine.[46] Following this self-removal, he reported experiencing a return of his taste sensation.[46] Once he refilled his prescription and began taking amlodipine a second time, his taste disturbance reoccurred.[46] These two cases suggest that there is an association between these drugs and taste disorders. This link is supported by the "de-challenge" and "re-challenge" that took place in both instances.[46] It appears that drug-induced dysgeusia can be alleviated by reducing the drug's dose or by substituting a second drug from the same class.[37]

Eprosartan.

Alpha lipoic acid

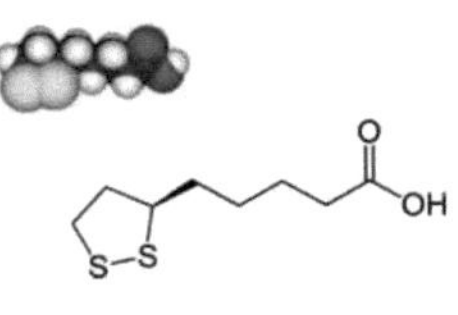

Alpha Lipoic Acid.

Alpha lipoic acid (ALA) is an antioxidant that is made naturally by human cells.[47] It can also be administered in capsules or can be found in foods such as red meat, organ meats, and yeast.[47] Like other antioxidants, it functions by ridding the body of harmful free radicals that can cause damage to tissues and organs.[47] It has an important role in the Krebs cycle as a coenzyme leading to the production of antioxidants, intracellular glutathione, and nerve-growth factors.[48] Animal research has also uncovered the ability of ALA to improve nerve conduction velocity.[48] Because flavors are perceived by differences in electric potential through specific nerves innervating the tongue, idiopathic dysgeusia may be a form of a neuropathy.[48] ALA has proven to be an effective treatment for burning mouth syndrome spurring studies in its potential to treat dysgeusia.[48] In a study of forty-four patients diagnosed with the disorder, one half was treated with the drug for two months while the other half, the control group, was given a placebo for two months followed by a two month treatment of ALA.[48] The results reported show that 91% of the group initially treated with ALA reported an improvement in their condition compared to only 36% of the control group.[48] After the control group was treated with ALA, 72% reported an improvement.[48] This study suggests that ALA may be a potential treatment for patients and supports that full double blind randomized studies should be performed.[48]

Managing dysgeusia

In addition to the aforementioned treatments, there are also many management approaches that can alleviate the symptoms of dysgeusia. These include using non-metallic silverware, avoiding metallic or bitter tasting foods, increasing the consumption of foods high in protein, flavoring foods with spices and seasonings, serving foods cold in order to reduce any unpleasant taste or odor, frequently brushing one's teeth and utilizing mouthwash, or using sialogogues such as chewing sugar-free gum or sour-tasting drops that stimulate the productivity of saliva.[41] When taste is impeded, the food experience can be improved through means other than taste, such as texture, aroma, temperature, and color.[44]

Psychological impacts

People who suffer from dysgeusia are also forced to manage the impact that the disorder has on their quality of life. An altered taste has effects on food choice and intake and can lead to weight loss, malnutrition, impaired immunity, and a decline in health.[44] Patients diagnosed with dysgeusia must use caution when adding sugar and salt to food and must be sure not to over compensate for their lack of taste with excess amounts.[44] Since the elderly are often on multiple medications, they are at risk for taste disturbances increasing the chances of developing depression, loss of appetite, and extreme weight loss.[49] This is cause for an evaluation and management of their dysgeusia. In patients undergoing chemotherapy, taste distortions can often be severe and make compliance with cancer treatment difficult.[42] Other problems that may arise include anorexia and behavioral changes that can be misinterpreted as psychiatric delusions regarding food.[50] Symptoms including paranoia, amnesia, cerebellar malfunction, and lethargy can also manifest when undergoing histidine treatment.[50] This makes it critical that these patients' dysgeusia is either treated or managed in order to improve their quality of life.

Future research

Every year, more than 200,000 individuals see their physicians concerning chemosensory problems, and many more taste disturbances are never reported.[51] Due to the large number of persons affected by taste disorders, basic and clinical research are receiving support at different institutions and chemosensory research centers across the country.[51] These taste and smell clinics are focusing their research on better understanding the mechanisms involved in gustatory function and taste disorders such as dysgeusia. For example, the National Institute on Deafness and Other Communication Disorders is looking into the mechanisms underlying the key receptors on taste cells and applying this knowledge to the future of medications and artificial food products.[51] Meanwhile, the Taste and Smell Clinic at the University of Connecticut Health Center is integrating behavioral, neurophysiological, and genetic studies involving stimulus concentrations and intensities in order to better understand taste function.[52] The purpose of these studies is to unearth the biological mechanisms underlying taste and to use this data to eliminate taste disorders in order to improve the lives of taste disorder sufferers.

See also

- Anosmia
- Parosmia

References

[1] http://apps.who.int/classifications/icd10/browse/2010/en#/R43.2

[2] http://www.icd9data.com/getICD9Code.ashx?icd9=781.1

[3] http://www.diseasesdatabase.com/ddb27369.htm

[4] http://www.nlm.nih.gov/medlineplus/ency/article/003050.htm

[5] http://www.emedicine.com/ent/topic333.htm

[6] Samuel K. Feske and Martin A. Samuels, *Office Practice of Neurology* 2nd ed. (Philadelphia: Elsevier Science, 2003)114.

[7] Norman M. Mann, MD, "Management of Smell and Taste Problems," *Cleveland Clinic Journal of Medicine* Apr. 2002: 334.

[8] Brand JG. Within reach of an end to unnecessary bitterness. Lancet. 2000;356:1371-1372.

[9] Beidler LM, Smallman RL. Renewal of cells within taste buds. J Cell Biol. 1965;27:263-272.

[10] Steven M. Bromley, MD, "Smell and Taste Disorders: A Primary Care Approach," *American Family Physician* 15 Jan 2000: 1.

[11] Masahide Yasuda and Hitoshi Tomita, "Electron Microscopic Observations of Glossal Circumvallate Papillae in Dysgeusic Patients," *Acta Otolaryngol* 2002: 126.

[12] Hoffman HJ, Ishii EK, MacTurk RH. Age-related changes in the prevalence of smell/taste problems among the United States adult population. Results of the 1994 disability supplement to the National Health Interview Survey (NHIS). Ann N Y Acad Sci. Nov 30 1998;855:716-22.

[13] Deems DA, Doty RL, Settle RG, et al. Smell and taste disorders: a study of 750 patients from the University of Pennsylvania Smell and Taste Center. Arch Otolaryngol Head Neck Surg. 1991;117:519-528.

[14] Hummel T, Knecht M. Smell and taste disorders. In: Calhoun KH, ed. Expert Guide to Otolaryngology. Philadelphia, Pa: American College of Physicians; 2001:650-664.

[15] Schiffman SS. Taste and smell in disease (first of two parts). N Engl J Med. 1983;308:1275-1279.

[16] Ahne G, Erras A, Hummel T, Kobal G. Assessment of gustatory function by means of tasting tablets. Laryngoscope. 2000;110:1396-1401.

[17] Seiden, Allen M., "Taste and Smell Disorders (Rhinology & Sinusology)," Thieme Publishing Group Aug. 2000: 153.

[18] Stillman JA, Morton RP, Goldsmith D. Automated electrogustometry: a new paradigm for the estimation of taste detection thresholds. Clin Otolaryngol. 2000;25:120-125.

[19] Murphy C, Quinonez C, Nordin S. Reliability and validity of electrogustometry and its application to young and elderly persons. Chem Senses. 1995;20:499-503.

[20] Jaaskelainen SK, Forssell H, Tenovuo O. Abnormalities of the blink reflex in burning mouth syndrome. Pain. 1997;73:455-460.

[21] Lell M, Schmid A, Stemper B, Maihöfner C, Heckmann JG, Tomandl BF. Simultaneous involvement of third and sixth cranial nerve in a patient with Lyme disease. Neuroradiology. 2003;45:85-87.

[22] Heckmann JG, Hilz MJ, Hummel T, et al. Oral mucosal blood flow following dry ice stimulation in humans. Clin Auton Res. 2000;10:317-321.

[23] Matsuo R. Role of saliva in the maintenance of taste sensitivity. Crit Rev Oral Biol Med. 2000;11:216-229.

[24] Robert I. Henkin, MD, PhD; Paul J. Schechter, MD, PhD; Robert Hoye, MD; Carl F. T. Mattern, MD. Idiopathic Hypogeusia With Dysgeusia, Hyposmia, and Dysosmia. JAMA. 1971;217(4):434-440.

[25] Judith E. Raber-Durlacher, Andrei Barasch, Douglas E. Peterson, Rajesh V. Lalla, Mark M. Schubert, and Willem E. Fibbe, "Oral Complications and Management Considerations in Patients Treated with High-Dosage Chemotherapy," *Supportive Cancer Therapy* Jul. 2004: 220.

[26] Micheal Wiseman, "The treatment of oral problems in the Palliative Patient," *Clinical Practice* Jun. 2006: 453.

[27] R. Matsuo, "Role of saliva in the maintenance of taste sensitivity," *Crit. Rev. Oral Biol. Med.*, 2000: 11.

[28] A. L. Speilman, "Interaction of Saliva and Taste," *J DENT RES*, 1990: 69.

[29] S. M. Heckmann, P. Hujoel, S. Habiger, W. Friess, M. Wichmann, J.G. Heckmann, and T. Hummel, "Zinc Gluconate in the treatment of Dysgeusia a Randomized Clinical Trial," *Journal of Dental Research* 2005: 37.

[30] Joseph M. Bicknell, MD and Robert V. Wiggins, MD, "Taste Disorder From Zinc Deficiency After Tonsillectomy," *The Western Journal of Medicine* Oct.1988: 458.

[31] F. Estelle R. Simmons, MD, "Advances in H1-Antihistamines," *The New England Journal of Medicine* 18 Nov. 2004: 2214.

[32] Samuel K. Feske and Martin A. Samuels, *Office Practice of Neurology* 2nd ed. (Philadelphia: Elsevier Science, 2003)119.

[33] Sebastian G. Ciancio, "Medications' impact on oral health," *Practical Science* Oct 2004: 1444.

[34] Xavier Castells, Isidre Rodoreda, Consuelo Pedrós, Gloria Cereza, and Joan-Ramon Laporte, "Drug Points," *BMJ* 30Nov 2002: 12777.

[35] R. K. Mal and M. A. Birchall, "Dysgeusia related to urinary obstruction from benign prostatic disease: a case control and qualitative study," *European Archives of Oto-Rhino Laryngology* 24 Aug. 2005:178.

[36] Giuseppe Lauria, Alessandra Majorana, Monica borgna, Raffaella Lombardi, Paola Penza, Alessandro padovani, and Pierluigi Sapelli, "Trigeminal small-fiber sensory neuropathy causes burning mouth syndrome," *Pain* 11 Mar. 2005: 332, 336.

[37] Giudice, Mirella, "Taste Disturbances Linked to Drug Use," *Canadian Pharmacist's Journal* Mar./Apr. 2006: 70.

[38] Preetha, A. and R. Banerjee, "Comparison of Artificial Saliva Substitutes, *Trends in Biomaterials and Artificial Organs*, Jan. 2005: 179.

[39] "Medications and Drugs," 6 May 2004, 25 Oct. 2009, <http://www.medicinenet.com/pilocarpine/article.htm>

[40] Heyneman, C., "Zinc Deficiency and Taste Disorders," *Ann Pharmacother*, Feb. 1996; 30(2): 186-187.

[41] Hong, Jae Hee, et al., "Taste and Odor Abnormalities in Cancer Patients," *The Journal of Supportive Oncology*, Mar./Apr. 2009: 59-64.

[42] Yamagata, T., et al., "The Pilot Trial of the Prevention of the Increase in Electrical Taste Thresholds by Zinc Containing Fluid Infusion during Chemotherapy to Treat Primary Lung Cancer," *Journal of Experimental and Clinical Cancer Research*, 2003; 22(4): 557.

[43] Halyard, Michele Y., "Taste and Smell Alterations in Cancer Patients- Real Problems With Few Solutions," *The Journal of Supportive Oncology*, Mar./Apr. 2009: 69.

[44] Bromley, Steven M., "Smell and Taste Disorders: A Primary Care Approach," American Family Physician 15 Jan. 2000, 23 Oct. 2009 <http://www.aafp.org/afp/20000115/427.html>

[45] Castells, Xavier, et al., "Drug Points: Dysgeusia and Burning Mouth Syndrome by Eprosartan," *British Medical Journal*, 30 Nov. 2002: 1277.

[46] Sadasivam, Balakrishnan and Ratinder Jhaj, "Dysgeusia with Amlodipine-a Case Report, *British Journal of Clinical Pharmacology*, 2006; 63(2): 253.

[47] University of Maryland Medical Center, "Alpha-lipoic Acid," 26 Oct. 2009 <http://www.umm.edu/altmed/articles/alpha-lipoic-000285.htm>

[48] Femiano, F., et al., "Idiopathic Dysgeusia; an Open Trial of Alpha Lipoic Acid (ALA) Therapy," *International Journal of Oral and Maxillofacial Surgery*, 2002; 31: 625-627.

[49] Padala, Kalpana, et al., "Mirtazapine Therapy for Dygeusia in the Elderly," *The Primary Care Companion to the Journal of Clinical Psychiatry*, 2006; 8(3): 178.

[50] Joseph M. Bicknell, MD and Robert V. Wiggins, MD, "Taste Disorder From Zinc Deficiency After Tonsillectomy," The Western Journal of Medicine Oct.1988: 458.

[51] National Institute on Deafness and Other Communication Disorders, "Taste Disorders," 25 June 2008, 23 Oct. 2009 <http://www.nidcd.nih.gov/health/smelltaste/taste.asp>

[52] The University of Connecticut Health Center, "Taste and Smell: Research," 26 Oct. 2009 <http://www.uchc.edu/uconntasteandsmell/research/index.html>

External links

- Dysgeusia at Yahoo! (http://health.yahoo.com/ency/healthwise/not257897)
- Dysgeusia at NIH (http://www.pubmedcentral.nih.gov/articlerender.fcgi?artid=1614219)

Subdural effusion

Subdural effusion	
Classification and external resources	
MeSH	D013353 [1]

Subdural effusion refers to an effusion in the subdural space, usually of cerebrospinal fluid. It is sometimes treated with surgery.[2]

References

[1] http://www.nlm.nih.gov/cgi/mesh/2011/MB_cgi?field=uid&term=D013353

[2] Yilmaz N, Kiymaz N, Yilmaz C, Bay A (2006). "Surgical treatment outcomes in subdural effusion: a clinical study" (http://content.karger. com/produktedb/produkte.asp?typ=fulltext&file=PNE2006042001001). *Pediatr Neurosurg* **42** (1): 1–3. doi:10.1159/000089502. PMID 16357494. .

See also

- Cerebrospinal fluid leak

Neurological disorders

A **neurological disorder** is a disorder of the body's nervous system. Structural, biochemical or electrical abnormalities in the brain, spinal cord or other nerves can result in a range of symptoms. Examples include paralysis, muscle weakness, poor coordination, loss of sensation, seizures, confusion, pain and altered levels of consciousness.There are many recognized neurological disorders, some relatively common, but many rare. They may be assessed by neurological examination, and studied and treated within the specialities of neurology and clinical neuropsychology. Examples of symptoms include

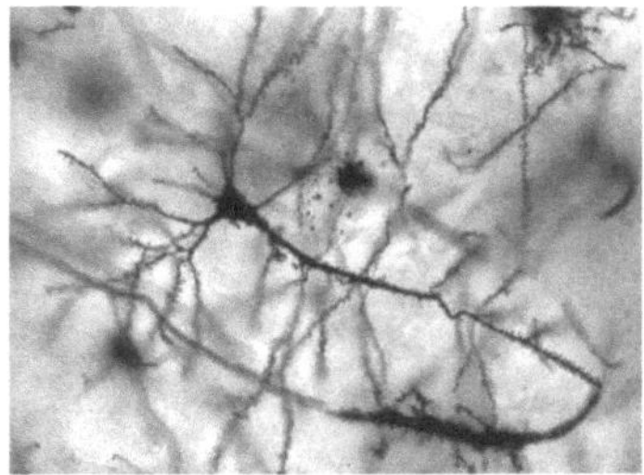

Neurons in patient with epilepsy, 40x magnified.

Interventions for neurological disorders include preventative measures, lifestyle changes, physiotherapy or other therapy, neurorehabilitation, pain management, medication, or operations performed by neurosurgeons. The World Health Organization estimated in 2006 that neurological disorders and their sequelae (direct consequences) affect as many as one billion people worldwide, and identified health inequalities and social stigma/discrimination as major factors contributing to the associated disability and suffering.[1]

Causes

Although the brain and spinal cord are surrounded by tough membranes, enclosed in the bones of the skull and spinal vertebrae, and chemically isolated by the so-called blood-brain barrier, they are very susceptible if compromised. Nerves tend to lie deep under the skin but can still become exposed to damage. Individual neurons, and the neural networks and nerves into which they form, are susceptible to electrochemical and structural disruption. Neuroregeneration may occur in the peripheral nervous system and thus overcome or work around injuries to some extent, it is thought to be rare in the brain and spinal cord.

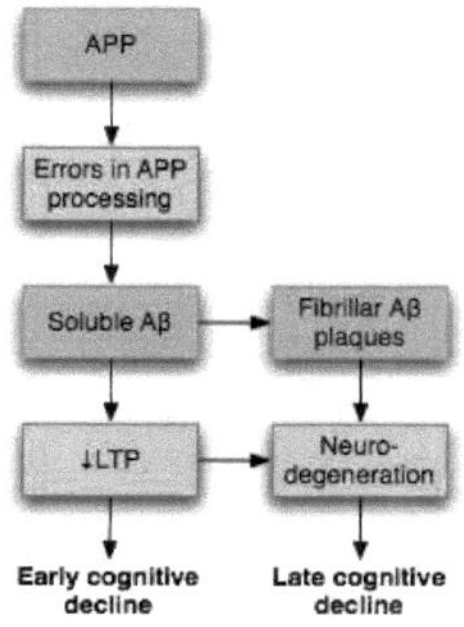

Part of the causal chain leading to Alzheimer's disease.

The specific causes of neurological problems vary, but can include genetic disorders; congenital abnormalities or disorders; infections; lifestyle or environmental health problems including malnutrition; and brain injury, spinal cord injury or nerve injury. The problem may start in another body system that interacts with the nervous system. For example, cerebrovascular disorders involve brain injury due to problems with the blood vessels (cardiovascular system) supplying the brain; autoimmune disorders involve damage caused by the body's own immune system; lysosomal storage diseases such as Niemann-Pick disease can lead to neurological deterioration.

In a substantial minority of cases of neurological symptoms, no neural cause can be identified using current testing procedures, and such "idiopathic" conditions can invite different theories about what is occurring.

Classification

Neurological disorders can be categorized according to the primary location affected, the primary type of dysfunction involved, or the primary type of cause. The broadest division is between central nervous system (CNS) disorders and peripheral nervous system (PNS) disorders. The Merck Manual lists brain, spinal cord and nerve disorders in the following overlapping categories:[2]

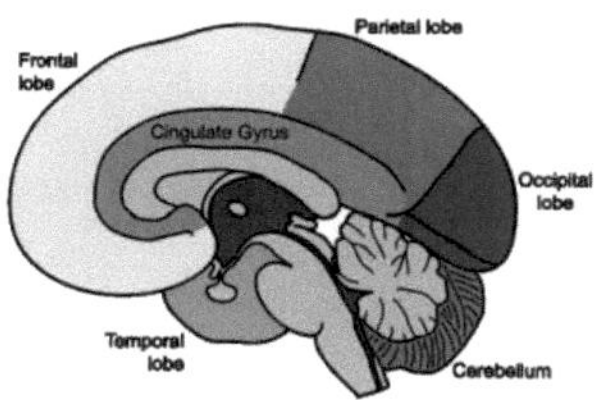

Anatomy of the human brain.

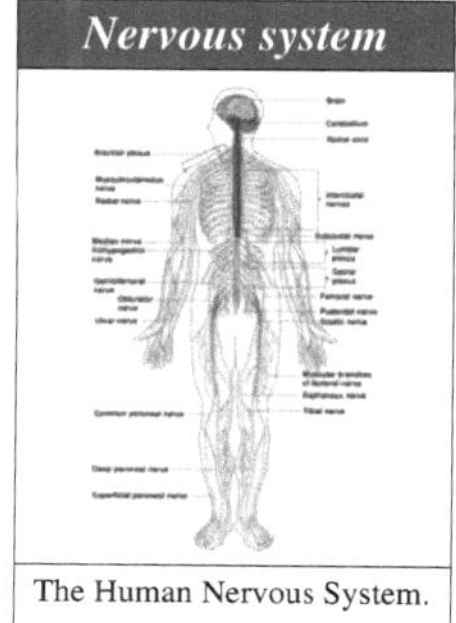

The Human Nervous System.

- Brain:
  - Brain damage according to cerebral lobe *(see also 'lower' brain areas such as basal ganglia, cerebellum, brainstem)*:
    - Frontal lobe damage
    - Parietal lobe damage
    - Temporal lobe damage
    - Occipital lobe damage
  - Brain dysfunction according to type:
    - Aphasia (language)
    - Dysarthria (speech)
    - Apraxia (patterns or sequences of movements)
    - Agnosia (identifying things/people)
    - Amnesia (memory)
- Spinal cord disorders (see spinal pathology, injury, inflammation)
- Peripheral nervous system disorders
- Cranial nerve disorders
- Autonomic nervous system disorders
- Seizure disorders such as epilepsy
- Movement disorders such as Parkinson's disease
- Sleep disorders
- Headaches (including migraine)
- Lower back and neck pain (see Back pain)
- Other pain (see Neuropathic pain)
- Delirium and dementia such as Alzheimer's disease
- Dizziness and vertigo
- Stupor and coma
- Head injury
- Stroke (CVA, cerebrovascular attack)
- Tumors of the nervous system (e.g. cancer)
- Multiple sclerosis (MS) and other demyelinating diseases
- Infections of the brain or spinal cord (including meningitis)
- Prion diseases (a type of infectious agent)
- Complex regional pain syndrome (CRPS) (a chronic pain condition.)

Neurological disorders in non-human animals are treated by veterinarians.[3] [4]

Mental functioning

A neurological examination can to some extent assess the impact of neurological damage and disease on brain function in terms of behavior, memory or cognition. Behavioral neurology specializes in this area. In addition, clinical neuropsychology uses neuropsychological assessment to precisely identify and track problems in mental functioning, usually after some sort of brain injury or neurological impairment.

Alternatively, a condition might first be detected through the presence of abnormalities in mental functioning, and further assessment may indicate an underlying neurological disorder. There are sometimes unclear boundaries in the distinction between disorders treated within neurology, and mental disorders treated within the other medical specialty of psychiatry, or other mental health professions such as clinical psychology. In practice, cases may present as one type but be assessed as more appropriate to the other.[5] neuropsychiatry deals with mental disorders arising from specific identified diseases of the nervous system.

One area that can be contested is in cases of idiopathic neurological symptoms - conditions where the cause cannot be established. It can be decided in some cases, perhaps by exclusion of any accepted diagnosis, that higher-level brain/mental activity is causing symptoms, rather than the symptoms originating in the area of the nervous system from which they may appear to originate. Classic examples are "functional" seizures, sensory numbness, "functional" limb weakness and functional neurological deficit ("functional" in this context is usually contrasted with the old term "organic disease"). Such cases may be contentiously interpreted as being "psychological" rather than "neurological". Some cases may be classified as mental disorders, for example as conversion disorder, if the symptoms appear to be causally linked to emotional states or responses to social stress or social contexts.

On the other hand, dissociation refer to partial or complete disruption of the integration of a person's conscious functioning, such that a person may feel detached from one's emotions, body and/or immediate surroundings. At one extreme this may be diagnosed as Depersonalization disorder. There are also conditions viewed as neurological where a person appears to consciously register neurological stimuli that cannot possibly be coming from the part of the nervous system to which they would normally be attributed, such as phantom pain or synesthesia, or where limbs act without conscious direction, as in alien hand syndrome. Theories and assumptions about consciousness, free will, Moral responsibility and social stigma can play a part in this, whether from the perspective of the clinician or the patient.

Conditions that are classed as mental disorders, or learning disabilities and forms of mental retardation, are not themselves usually dealt with as neurological disorders. Biological psychiatry seeks to understand mental disorders in terms of their basis in the nervous system, however. In clinical practice, mental disorders are usually indicated by a mental state examination, or other type of structured interview or questionnaire process. At the present time, neuroimaging (brain scans) alone cannot accurately diagnose a mental disorder or tell the risk of developing one; however, it can be used to rule out other medical conditions such as a brain tumor.[6] In research, neuroimaging and other neurological tests can show correlations between reported and observed mental difficulties and certain aspects of neural function or differences in brain structure. In general, numerous fields intersect to try and understand the basic processes involved in mental functioning,

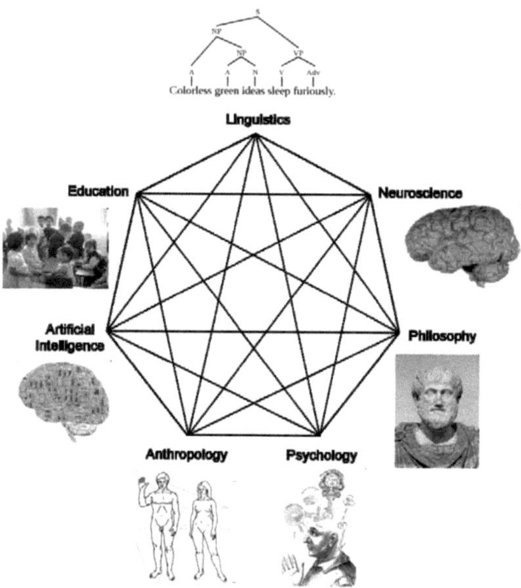

Different levels of analysis in the understanding of mental functioning.

many of which are brought together in cognitive science. The distinction between neurological and mental disorders can be a matter of some debate, either in regard to specific facts about the cause of a condition or in regard to the general understanding of brain and mind.

Moveover, the definition of disorder in medicine or psychology is sometimes contested in terms of what is considered abnormal, dysfunctional, harmful or unnatural in neurological, evolutionary, psychometric or social terms.

See also

- Central nervous system
- Peripheral nervous system
- Human brain
- ICD-10 Chapter VI: Diseases of the nervous system
- Mental disorder
- Neuroplasticity

External links

- Disorder Index [7] of the National Institute of Neurological Disorders and Stroke

References

[1] WHO Neurological Disorders: Public Health Challenges (http://www.who.int/mental_health/neurology/neurodiso/en/index.html)

[2] Merck Manual: Brain, Spinal Cord and Nerve Disorders (http://www.merck.com/mmhe/sec06.html)

[3] Veterinary Neurological Centre - Neurological Signs and Diseases (http://www.vetneuro.com/NeurologicalSignsDiseases/tabid/4171/Default.aspx)

[4] Merck Veterinary Manual - Nervous System (http://www.merckvetmanual.com/mvm/index.jsp?cfile=htm/bc/toc_100000.htm)

[5] Butler, C (1 March 2005). "Neurological syndromes which can be mistaken for psychiatric conditions" (http://jnnp.bmj.com/content/76/suppl_1/i31.full). *Journal of Neurology, Neurosurgery & Psychiatry* **76** (suppl_1): i31–i38. doi:10.1136/jnnp.2004.060459. .

[6] NIMH publications (2009) Neuroimaging and Mental Illness (http://www.nimh.nih.gov/health/publications/neuroimaging-and-mental-illness-a-window-into-the-brain/neuroimaging-and-mental-illness-a-window-into-the-brain.shtml)

[7] http://www.ninds.nih.gov/disorders/disorder_index.htm

Article Sources and Contributors

Spontaneous cerebrospinal fluid leak *Source*: http://en.wikipedia.org/w/index.php?title=Spontaneous_cerebrospinal_fluid_leak *Contributors*: 0kmck4gmja, Arcadian, ArnoldReinhold, AugPi, Axl, Basket of Puppies, BurtAlert, Delldot, Diego Grez, DragonflySixtyseven, Ebikeguy, Elen of the Roads, Foolsgold55, Fuhghettaboutit, Gaius Cornelius, Garrondo, Graham87, Gurch, H1nkles, Hamtechperson, Hersfold, JHiesey, Jfdwolff, Jmh649, Joel7687, Jwy, Khazar, Koavf, Kumioko, L'Aquatique, LinguistAtLarge, Lmrke4415, Maralia, Mild Bill Hiccup, Mm40, Mr etler, NativeForeigner, NocturneNoir, Nono64, Shirik, Sonia, Stevenfruitsmaak, Sven Manguard, The Anome, Tide rolls, Timotheus Canens, Tpbradbury, Vaizdu, Wackywace, Whiteguru, Zscout370, 17 anonymous edits

Cerebrospinal fluid *Source*: http://en.wikipedia.org/w/index.php?title=Cerebrospinal_fluid *Contributors*: 63.86.107.xxx, Ace111, Aceofhearts1968, Amaher, Antifumo, ApersOn, Arc de Ciel, Arcadian, Basket of Puppies, Bissinger, Bobo192, Bryan Derksen, CDN99, Cai, Cerejota, Cezarika1, Chidicon, Cmcnicoll, Conversion script, Cool faces, CorporalW, Dlohcierekim, Dnwq, DocWatson42, Dr. St-Amant, Drphilharmonic, Edgar181, Emperorbma, Eras-mus, ErdemTuzun, Fadliabdullah, Fantumphool, Gadlen, Gaius Cornelius, Giancarlo Rossi, Gilliam, Ginkgo100, Gouerouz, Graham87, Gromlakh, Hede2000, Herbythyme, IdealOmniscience, Immunize, Irutavias, JackWasey, Jauhienij, Jcoakes9, Jeffq, JeremyA, Jfdwolff, Jimp, Jlmoltzen, Jmacaulay, Jmh649, Joehall45, Kenn03, Kosigrim, Kruosio, Lipothymia, Looie496, Luke poa, Mav, Maxxicum, Merenta, Mesoderm, Mikael Häggström, Moltovivace, N5iln, Nassim Abi Chahine, Neutrality, Nevit, NickCT, Nickkid5, Nicksh, Nivekian, Nohomers48, Nono64, NotWith, Nunh-huh, Nyttend, OohBunnies!, Perfectapproach, Permacultura, PrestonH, Quarl, R107, RLeopard, Rashka00, Reza luke, Rjwilmsi, Rockithegreat, Romanm, S7evyn, Saariko, Sbmehta, Shameerbabu986, Sjschen, Smjg, Spitfire, Srikeit, Tarotcards, Tarsaucer, The Thing That Should Not Be, Theolyons, Timwi, Tobias Hoevekamp, Tomaxer, Tri6ky, TurtleShroom, Ugur Basak, Vojtech.dostal, Wdustbuster, WereSpielChequers, White Trillium, Whiteknight, Wisdom89, WolfmanSF, Woohookitty, Wouterhagens, Wouterstomp, Wyvyrn, Zeus1234, Ziphon, 180 anonymous edits

Dura mater *Source*: http://en.wikipedia.org/w/index.php?title=Dura_mater *Contributors*: A314268, Alex.tan, Anatomist90, Andris, Annekcm, Arcadian, Asml8d, Basket of Puppies, Bemoeial, Bryan Derksen, Carrionluggage, Chirality, Claudication, Cmcnicoll, Deflective, Dekimasu, Delldot, Diberri, DrFO.Jr.Tn, Dreviscerator, Drgarden, Drift chambers, ErikvanB, Gaius Cornelius, Giftlite, Hehkuviini, IVIoI3iuS, JForget, Japanese Searobin, Jfurr1981, Keenan Pepper, KieferSkunk, Kimnn, Kwamikagami, La goutte de pluie, Ljfa-ag, Lmjohns3, MVillani1985, Mikael Häggström, Moormand, Mysid, Neko-chan, Obaid221, Onco p53, PhatRita, Pwjb, Rbklassen, Rembecki, Riyehn, SalvoIsaja, Schmloof, Selket, SkyMaja, Snowmanradio, The Anome, Tide rolls, Zyryab, 61 anonymous edits

Meninges *Source*: http://en.wikipedia.org/w/index.php?title=Meninges *Contributors*: Adammathias, Alex.tan, Algumacoisaqq, ApersOn, Arcadian, BrOnXbOmBr21, Bryan Derksen, CanisRufus, Chefyingi, DTM, DeadEyeArrow, Delldot, Delldot on a public computer, Dethomas, DrFO.Jr.Tn, DrJos, Drgarden, Emperorbma, EncycloPetey, Exert, Gadriel, Gludwiczak, Gouerouz, Habj, HobbesPDX, Iridescent, Jeffq, Jfdwolff, Joehall45, Jonkerz, Junglecat, KellyCoinGuy, Krishnan2424, L Kensington, Lova Falk, Macedonian, Madhero88, Mashford, Mayteng, Mild Bill Hiccup, Mimihitam, Montrealais, Mysid, N3bulous, NellieBly, NightWolf1298, Nono64, Nwbeeson, Paiamshadi, PhatRita, Rlue, RodC, Saaga, Sayeth, Selket, Shatrughansingh77116, Shawn in Montreal, SwisterTwister, Tanjx, Tellyaddict, The Thing That Should Not Be, Tim Q. Wells, Tristanb, Vedran12, Wisebridge, Wouterstomp, 95 anonymous edits

Cerebrospinal fluid leak *Source*: http://en.wikipedia.org/w/index.php?title=Cerebrospinal_fluid_leak *Contributors*: Acdx, Arcadian, Basket of Puppies, Jfdwolff, LinguistAtLarge, MoonMan, 4 anonymous edits

Idiopathic *Source*: http://en.wikipedia.org/w/index.php?title=Idiopathic *Contributors*: Alan Liefting, Alessandro f2001, Alteripse, Anthonyhcole, Arteitle, Belchman, Belljaf, Biscuittin, Boing! said Zebedee, Bryankennedy, Colin, Cornellrockey, Craverguy, DRosenbach, Dah31, DavidWBrooks, Diberri, Doc Mike, Dougie monty, Dresdnhope, Ellywa, Grendelkhan, Holothurion, Jbublick, Jclerman, Jfdwolff, Jmarchn, Jmjanzen, Jonboy01, Kizor, Kubanczyk, Lazarus1907, Le Anh-Huy, Lysy, MPerel, MarcoTolo, Mendalus, Moshe Constantine Hassan Al-Silverburg, Nigholith, Phschink, Power.corrupts, Purpleturple, Rbh00, Rentar, Richard Arthur Norton (1958-), Saga City, SidP, Steno55, Tarek, TimVickers, Tsemii, Vicarious, Vogon77, WalkinDownThirtyThree, Wasell, Zaakuru808, 47 anonymous edits

Facial weakness *Source*: http://en.wikipedia.org/w/index.php?title=Facial_weakness *Contributors*: Arcadian, AugPi, Bearcat, Crystallina, FSHSOCIETY, Salah Almhamdi, Woodsstock, Xezbeth

Epidural blood patch *Source*: http://en.wikipedia.org/w/index.php?title=Epidural_blood_patch *Contributors*: 0kmck4gmja, Almazi, Betacommand, Cantons-de-l'Est, CliffC, CommonsDelinker, Graham87, Kosebamse, L'Aquatique, Oddharmonic, Wouterstomp, 9 anonymous edits

Georg Schaltenbrand *Source*: http://en.wikipedia.org/w/index.php?title=Georg_Schaltenbrand *Contributors*: Diego Grez, Gabbe, Plindenbaum, Postcard Cathy, Waacstats, 1 anonymous edits

Spinal canal *Source*: http://en.wikipedia.org/w/index.php?title=Spinal_canal *Contributors*: ABF, Al Lemos, Anthonyhcole, Arcadian, Barzkar, Bibi Saint-Pol, Bogey97, Caerwine, Creidieki, Eleassar, Hadal, Joyous!, Kohhei, Mark Richards, Mikael Häggström, Mmrruugg, Mysid, Rich Farmbrough, Scottalter, Tomas e, Xiaop, יסמ, 10 anonymous edits

Orthostatic headache *Source*: http://en.wikipedia.org/w/index.php?title=Orthostatic_headache *Contributors*: Basket of Puppies, Bunnyhop11, GregorB, 1 anonymous edits

Dysgeusia *Source*: http://en.wikipedia.org/w/index.php?title=Dysgeusia *Contributors*: Aranel, Arbitrarily0, Arcadian, Auntof6, Beland, Belovedfreak, Bobber0001, C6541, CDN99, Chengkd, Crystallina, Cybercobra, Danielil, Deflective, Dylan620, Eritain, Fragileartofexistence, Gandhi7, Intelati, JamesAM, Jncraton, Johnkarp, Katie1341, KrakatoaKatie, KungFuRealTalk, Kwamikagami, LilHelpa, M.e, Notheruser, SchreiberBike, Simplepink, Tim Q. Wells, WLU, Wantsarevolution, William Avery, רור55, 26 anonymous edits

Subdural effusion *Source*: http://en.wikipedia.org/w/index.php?title=Subdural_effusion *Contributors*: Arcadian, Shire Reeve

Neurological disorders *Source*: http://en.wikipedia.org/w/index.php?title=Neurological_disorders *Contributors*: Aaron Kauppi, Alansohn, Angela, Anthonyhcole, Arcadian, Cold Season, Erich gasboy, EverSince, Gadfium, Graham87, Helmoony, Ida Shaw, Immunize, Jfdwolff, John of Reading, Jonkerz, Kirkus M, Leevanjackson, MZMcBride, Magnus Manske, Mav, Niceguyedc, Nihiltres, Nono64, Paulbmann, Philip Trueman, PierreAbbat, Pile-Up, R'n'B, R500Mom, RedWolf, Tbhotch, True Pagan Warrior, Tweak279, Vicki Rosenzweig, Zigger, 20 anonymous edits

Image Sources, Licenses and Contributors

GNU Free Documentation License Version 1.2, November 2002

0. PREAMBLE

The purpose of this License is to make a manual, textbook, or other functional and useful document "free" in the sense of freedom: to assure everyone the effective freedom to copy and redistribute it, with or without modifying it, either commercially or noncommercially. Secondarily, this License preserves for the author and publisher a way to get credit for their work, while not being considered responsible for modifications made by others. This License is a kind of "copyleft", which means that derivative works of the document must themselves be free in the same sense. It complements the GNU General Public License, which is a copyleft license designed for free software. We have designed this License in order to use it for manuals for free software, because free software needs free documentation: a free program should come with manuals providing the same freedoms that the software does. But this License is not limited to software manuals; it can be used for any textual work, regardless of subject matter or whether it is published as a printed book. We recommend this License principally for works whose purpose is instruction or reference.

1. APPLICABILITY AND DEFINITIONS

This License applies to any manual or other work, in any medium, that contains a notice placed by the copyright holder saying it can be distributed under the terms of this License. Such a notice grants a world-wide, royalty-free license, unlimited in duration, to use that work under the conditions stated herein. The "Document", below, refers to any such manual or work. Any member of the public is a licensee, and is addressed as "you". You accept the license if you copy, modify or distribute the work in a way requiring permission under copyright law. A "Modified Version" of the Document means any work containing the Document or a portion of it, either copied verbatim, or with modifications and/or translated into another language. A "Secondary Section" is a named appendix or a front-matter section of the Document that deals exclusively with the relationship of the publishers or authors of the Document to the Document's overall subject (or to related matters) and contains nothing that could fall directly within that overall subject. (Thus, if the Document is in part a textbook of mathematics, a Secondary Section may not explain any mathematics.) The relationship could be a matter of historical connection with the subject or with related matters, or of legal, commercial, philosophical, ethical or political position regarding them. The "Invariant Sections" are certain Secondary Sections whose titles are designated, as being those of Invariant Sections, in the notice that says that the Document is released under this License. If a section does not fit the above definition of Secondary then it is not allowed to be designated as Invariant. The Document may contain zero Invariant Sections. If the Document does not identify any Invariant Sections then there are none. The "Cover Texts" are certain short passages of text that are listed, as Front-Cover Texts or Back-Cover Texts, in the notice that says that the Document is released under this License. A Front-Cover Text may be at most 5 words, and a Back-Cover Text may be at most 25 words. A "Transparent" copy of the Document means a machine-readable copy, represented in a format whose specification is available to the general public, that is suitable for revising the document straightforwardly with generic text editors or (for images composed of pixels) generic paint programs or (for drawings) some widely available drawing editor, and that is suitable for input to text formatters or for automatic translation to a variety of formats suitable for input to text formatters. A copy made in an otherwise Transparent file format whose markup, or absence of markup, has been arranged to thwart or discourage subsequent modification by readers is not Transparent. An image format is not Transparent if used for any substantial amount of text. A copy that is not "Transparent" is called "Opaque". Examples of suitable formats for Transparent copies include plain ASCII without markup, Texinfo input format, LaTeX input format, SGML or XML using a publicly available DTD, and standard-conforming simple HTML, PostScript or PDF designed for human modification. Examples of transparent image formats include PNG, XCF and JPG. Opaque formats include proprietary formats that can be read and edited only by proprietary word processors, SGML or XML for which the DTD and/or processing tools are not generally available, and the machine-generated HTML, PostScript or PDF produced by some word processors for output purposes only. The "Title Page" means, for a printed book, the title page itself, plus such following pages as are needed to hold, legibly, the material this License requires to appear in the title page. For works in formats which do not have any title page as such, "Title Page" means the text near the most prominent appearance of the work's title, preceding the beginning of the body of the text. A section "Entitled XYZ" means a named subunit of the Document whose title either is precisely XYZ or contains XYZ in parentheses following text that translates XYZ in another language. (Here XYZ stands for a specific section name mentioned below, such as "Acknowledgements", "Dedications", "Endorsements", or "History".) To "Preserve the Title" of such a section when you modify the Document means that it remains a section "Entitled XYZ" according to this definition. The Document may include Warranty Disclaimers next to the notice which states that this License applies to the Document. These Warranty Disclaimers are considered to be included by reference in this License, but only as regards disclaiming warranties: any other implication that these Warranty Disclaimers may have is void and has no effect on the meaning of this License.

2. VERBATIM COPYING

You may copy and distribute the Document in any medium, either commercially or noncommercially, provided that this License, the copyright notices, and the license notice saying this License applies to the Document are reproduced in all copies, and that you add no other conditions whatsoever to those of this License. You may not use technical measures to obstruct or control the reading or further copying of the copies you make or distribute. However, you may accept compensation in exchange for copies. If you distribute a large enough number of copies you must also follow the conditions in section 3. You may also lend copies, under the same conditions stated above, and you may publicly display copies.

3. COPYING IN QUANTITY

If you publish printed copies (or copies in media that commonly have printed covers) of the Document, numbering more than 100, and the Document's license notice requires Cover Texts, you must enclose the copies in covers that carry, clearly and legibly, all these Cover Texts: Front-Cover Texts on the front cover, and Back-Cover Texts on the back cover. Both covers must also clearly and legibly identify you as the publisher of these copies. The front cover must present the full title with all words of the title equally prominent and visible. You may add other material on the covers in addition. Copying with changes limited to the covers, as long as they preserve the title of the Document and satisfy these conditions, can be treated as verbatim copying in other respects. If the required texts for either cover are too voluminous to fit legibly, you should put the first ones listed (as many as fit reasonably) on the actual cover, and continue the rest onto adjacent pages. If you publish or distribute Opaque copies of the Document numbering more than 100, you must either include a machine-readable Transparent copy along with each Opaque copy, or state in or with each Opaque copy a computer-network location from which the general network-using public has access to download using public-standard network protocols a complete Transparent copy of the Document, free of added material. If you use the latter option, you must take reasonably prudent steps, when you begin distribution of Opaque copies in quantity, to ensure that this Transparent copy will remain thus accessible at the stated location until at least one year after the last time you distribute an Opaque copy (directly or through your agents or retailers) of that edition to the public. It is requested, but not required, that you contact the authors of the Document well before redistributing any large number of copies, to give them a chance to provide you with an updated version of the Document.

4. MODIFICATIONS

You may copy and distribute a Modified Version of the Document under the conditions of sections 2 and 3 above, provided that you release the Modified Version under precisely this License, with the Modified Version filling the role of the Document, thus licensing distribution and modification of the Modified Version to whoever possesses a copy of it. In addition, you must do these things in the Modified Version: A. Use in the Title Page (and on the covers, if any) a title distinct from that of the Document, and from those of previous versions (which should, if there were any, be listed in the History section of the Document). You may use the same title as a previous version if the original publisher of that version gives permission. B. List on the Title Page, as authors, one or more persons or entities responsible for authorship of the modifications in the Modified Version, together with at least five of the principal authors of the Document (all of its principal authors, if it has fewer than five), unless they release you from this requirement. C. State on the Title page the name of the publisher of the Modified Version, as the publisher. D. Preserve all the copyright notices of the Document. E. Add an appropriate copyright notice for your modifications adjacent to the other copyright notices. F. Include, immediately after the copyright notices, a license notice giving the public permission to use the Modified Version under the terms of this License, in the form shown in the Addendum below. G. Preserve in that license notice the full lists of Invariant Sections and required Cover Texts given in the Document's license notice. H. Include an unaltered copy of this License. I. Preserve the section Entitled "History", Preserve its Title, and add to it an item stating at least the title, year, new authors, and publisher of the Modified Version as given on the Title Page. If there is no section Entitled "History" in the Document, create one stating the title, year, authors, and publisher of the Document as given on its Title Page, then add an item describing the Modified Version as stated in the previous sentence. J. Preserve the network location, if any, given in the Document for public access to a Transparent copy of the Document, and likewise the network locations given in the Document for previous versions it was based on. These may be placed in the "History" section. You may omit a network location for a work that was published at least four years before the Document itself, or if the original publisher of the version it refers to gives permission. K. For any section Entitled "Acknowledgements" or "Dedications", Preserve the Title of the section, and preserve in the section all the substance and tone of each of the contributor acknowledgements and/or dedications given therein. L. Preserve all the Invariant Sections of the Document, unaltered in their text and in their titles. Section numbers or the equivalent are not considered part of the section titles. M. Delete any section Entitled "Endorsements". Such a section may not be included in the Modified Version. N. Do not retitle any existing section to be Entitled "Endorsements" or to conflict in title with any Invariant Section. O. Preserve any Warranty Disclaimers. If the Modified Version includes new front-matter sections or appendices that qualify as Secondary Sections and contain no material copied from the Document, you may at your option designate some or all of these sections as invariant. To do this, add their titles to the list of Invariant Sections in the Modified Version's license notice. These titles must be distinct from any other section titles. You may add a section Entitled "Endorsements", provided it contains nothing but endorsements of your Modified Version by various parties--for example, statements of peer review or that the text has been approved by an organization as the authoritative definition of a standard. You may add a passage of up to five words as a Front-Cover Text, and a passage of up to 25 words as a Back-Cover Text, to the end of the list of Cover Texts in the Modified Version. Only one passage of Front-Cover Text and one of Back-Cover Text may be added by (or through arrangements made by) any one entity. If the Document already includes a cover text for the same cover, previously added by you or by arrangement made by the same entity you are acting on behalf of, you may not add another; but you may replace the old one, on explicit permission from the previous publisher that added the old one. The author(s) and publisher(s) of the Document do not by this License give permission to use their names for publicity for or to assert or imply endorsement of any Modified Version.

5. COMBINING DOCUMENTS

You may combine the Document with other documents released under this License, under the terms defined in section 4 above for modified versions, provided that you include in the combination all of the Invariant Sections of all of the original documents, unmodified, and list them all as Invariant Sections of your combined work in its license notice, and that you preserve all their Warranty Disclaimers. The combined work need only contain one copy of this License, and multiple identical Invariant Sections may be replaced with a single copy. If there are multiple Invariant Sections with the same name but different contents, make the title of each such section unique by adding at the end of it, in parentheses, the name of the original author or publisher of that section if known, or else a unique number. Make the same adjustment to the section titles in the list of Invariant Sections in the license notice of the combined work. In the combination, you must combine any sections Entitled "History" in the various original documents, forming one section Entitled "History"; likewise combine any sections Entitled "Acknowledgements", and any sections Entitled "Dedications". You must delete all sections Entitled "Endorsements".

6. COLLECTIONS OF DOCUMENTS

You may make a collection consisting of the Document and other documents released under this License, and replace the individual copies of this License in the various documents with a single copy that is included in the collection, provided that you follow the rules of this License for verbatim copying of each of the documents in all other respects. You may extract a single document from such a collection, and distribute it individually under this License, provided you insert a copy of this License into the extracted document, and follow this License in all other respects regarding verbatim copying of that document.

7. AGGREGATION WITH INDEPENDENT WORKS

A compilation of the Document or its derivatives with other separate and independent documents or works, in or on a volume of a storage or distribution medium, is called an "aggregate" if the copyright resulting from the compilation is not used to limit the legal rights of the compilation's users beyond what the individual works permit. When the Document is included in an aggregate, this License does not apply to the other works in the aggregate which are not themselves derivative works of the Document. If the Cover Text requirement of section 3 is applicable to these copies of the Document, then if the Document is less than one half of the entire aggregate, the Document's Cover Texts may be placed on covers that bracket the Document within the aggregate, or the electronic equivalent of covers if the Document is in electronic form. Otherwise they must appear on printed covers that bracket the whole aggregate.

8. TRANSLATION

Translation is considered a kind of modification, so you may distribute translations of the Document under the terms of section 4. Replacing Invariant Sections with translations requires special permission from their copyright holders, but you may include translations of some or all Invariant Sections in addition to the original versions of these Invariant Sections. You may include a translation of this License, and all the license notices in the Document, and any Warranty Disclaimers, provided that you also include the original English version of this License and the original versions of those notices and disclaimers. In case of a disagreement between the translation and the original version of this License or a notice or disclaimer, the original version will prevail. If a section in the Document is Entitled "Acknowledgements", "Dedications", or "History", the requirement (section 4) to Preserve its Title (section 1) will typically require changing the actual title.

9. TERMINATION

You may not copy, modify, sublicense, or distribute the Document except as expressly provided for under this License. Any other attempt to copy, modify, sublicense or distribute the Document is void, and will automatically terminate your rights under this License. However, parties who have received copies, or rights, from you under this License will not have their licenses terminated so long as such parties remain in full compliance.

10. FUTURE REVISIONS OF THIS LICENSE

The Free Software Foundation may publish new, revised versions of the GNU Free Documentation License from time to time. Such new versions will be similar in spirit to the present version, but may differ in detail to address new problems or concerns. See http://www.gnu.org/copyleft/. Each version of the License is given a distinguishing version number. If the Document specifies that a particular numbered version of this License "or any later version" applies to it, you have the option of following the terms and conditions either of that specified version or of any later version that has been published (not as a draft) by the Free Software Foundation. If the Document does not specify a version number of this License, you may choose any version ever published (not as a draft) by the Free Software Foundation. ADDENDUM: How to use this License for your documents To use this License in a document you have written, include a copy of the License in the document and put the following copyright and license notices just after the title page: Copyright (c) YEAR YOUR NAME. Permission is granted to copy, distribute and/or modify this document under the terms of the GNU Free Documentation License, Version 1.2 or any later version published by the Free Software Foundation; with no Invariant Sections, no Front-Cover Texts, and no Back-Cover Texts. A copy of the license is included in the section entitled "GNU Free Documentation License". If you have Invariant Sections, Front-Cover Texts and Back-Cover Texts, replace the "with...Texts." line with this: with the Invariant Sections being LIST THEIR TITLES, with the Front-Cover Texts being LIST, and with the Back-Cover Texts being LIST. If you have Invariant Sections without Cover Texts, or some other combination of the three, merge those two alternatives to suit the situation. If your document contains nontrivial examples of program code, we recommend releasing these examples in parallel under your choice of free software license, such as the GNU General Public License, to permit their use in free software.

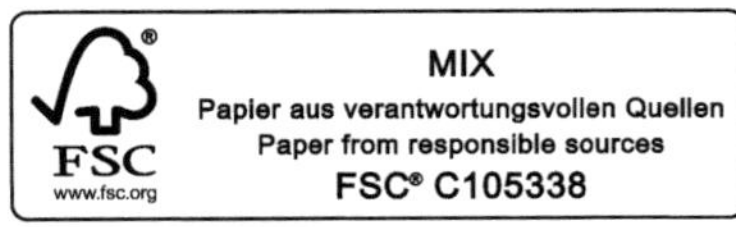

Printed by Books on Demand GmbH, Norderstedt / Germany